ENCYCLOPEDIA OF FAMILY HEALTH & WELLNESS

Volume 5   I–L

Table of Contents

How to Use This Book 6

How to Use the Interactive CDs 7

Introduction 8

I
Immune System 11
Immunization 16
Impotence 17
Incontinence 18
Indigestion 20
Infection and Infectious Diseases 20
Infectious Mononucleosis 26
Infertility 28
Influenza 28
Inhalants 31
Insomnia 33
Insulin 34
Internal Examination 35
Intestines 36
Intoxication 37
In Vitro Fertilization 39
Irritable Bowel Syndrome 39
Itches 39

J
Jaundice 41
Joints 42

K
Kidneys 46
Knee 48

L
Lacerations 49
Lactation 49
Larynx and Laryngitis 50
Lasers 51
LASIK Surgery 53
Laxatives 53
Lead Poisoning 54
Learning Disabilities 55
Leukemia 57
Life Expectancy 63
Ligaments 64
Liposuction 65
Liver 65
Local Anesthetics 68
Lower-Back Pain 68
LSD 70
Lungs 72
Lyme Disease 75
Lymphatic System 78

Glossary of Health Terms 82

Learn More 86

Index 92

Author Biography 96

How to Use This Book

We all have questions, concerns, and occasional fears about our health; we all wonder if we're doing all we should to keep our families and ourselves healthy. Sometimes, though, it's hard to even find the right words to shape our questions. This book and the other volumes in the *Encyclopedia of Family Health & Wellness* will help you answer some of the questions you might feel uncomfortable asking your doctor. It will also give you the understanding to know some of the questions you should ask and how to ask them more knowledgeably.

Keep in mind, though, that no book can ever take the place of health-care professionals. As the old saying goes, the person who doctors himself has a fool for a doctor! Only a trained medical provider can diagnose and treat illnesses. By the same token, the first-aid information contained in these volumes should never replace taking a certified first-aid course.

These books, however, can help you to:

- better understand what others are experiencing (for instance, if a family member has cancer or if a friend has allergies).
- learn more about your own body and how to keep it healthy.
- get ideas for school projects.
- find reliable sources for more in-depth research on particular topics.

Information is offered in easy-to-read, short entries, with highlighted terms included in each entry to guide you to topics found elsewhere in the encyclopedia. The "Learn More" section at the back of each volume and the Web sites included at the end of many of the entries direct you to additional information on the various topics. The glossary in the back of these books will also provide an introduction to some basic health terms and concepts that will be important for understanding the encyclopedia better.

Use these books in your home library, in health classes, in doctors' offices, and in school libraries. But always remember: never use them to replace the advice of a trained medical professional!

How to Use the Interactive CDs

In today's electronic world, many young people (and adults, too) are more comfortable with digital versions of print material. The *Encyclopedia of Family Health & Wellness* includes two CDs to supplement the text volumes.

The first of these is a linked and searchable version of the print text. This CD allows you to quickly find all references to a given topic, anywhere in the 10 volumes; it also enables users to jump back and forth between the linked subentries. In addition, the CD gives you the option of putting the text on your personal computer for ready access.

The second CD is a supplement that provides additional information on the following topics:

- the human body
- nutrition and exercise
- first aid and emergencies
- illness and disease

The sections that cover these topics each contain interactive images that will appeal to all ages. There are coloring pages for younger students and family members, and for older children, there are word searches, fill-in-the blank quizzes, and drag-and-drop games. The interactive CD encourages learning, promotes health and wellness in young people, and improves computer skills.

Don't forget: the information on these CDs, like the information in the printed books, should never replace the advice of trained health-care providers, nor should the first-aid information be considered a replacement for a certified course.

Introduction

What does it mean to be healthy?

It's the sort of word we all assume we understand—but in recent years, its meaning may have become more complex than it once was. The World Health Organization (WHO), for example, defines health as "a state of complete physical, mental, and social well-being, not merely the absence of disease or infirmity." In other words, a healthy person is not simply one who isn't sick; a healthy person feels well physically, thinks clearly, and gets along with others. This person's body, mind, and social interactions are all functioning at their optimum level. As author James H. West said,

Health is a large word. It embraces not the body only, but the mind and spirit as well . . . and not today's pain or pleasure alone, but the whole being and outlook.

When we think in these multifaceted terms, health may seem like a near-impossible goal to achieve. Our parents and grandparents were familiar with simple health proverbs such as "An apple a day keeps the doctor away," and "Early to bed, early to rise, makes a man healthy, wealthy, and wise." Today we still recognize the connections between health and diet and sleep—but we've also become aware of many more complicated interactions between the environment, our behaviors, and our health. How do we sort through the many issues that have an impact on our well-being?

The answers to this question will never be simple. Some of the circumstances that affect our health, such as genetics and global environmental issues, are beyond our control. Others, however, have more to do with lifestyle choices, things that are, in fact, up to us. Most health factors are actually interconnected, a complicated web of genetics, environment, and individual actions. The more we understand the many elements of wellness, the greater will be our ability to make wise choices.

That's what the 10 volumes in the *Encyclopedia of Family Health & Wellness* offer you—practical information you and your family can use to build healthy lifestyles. The more you know, the more power you have over your own well-being.

This solid foundation of practical knowledge is particularly important at the family level, where daily habits build the structure of an overall lifestyle. Parents are not the only ones who make important decisions affecting the family's health. Even the youngest members of the family can benefit from integrating health information into their knowledge base. Within the home—that framework of routines and expectations, as well as structural walls—the family exists as a living organism where the well-being of each member is linked to every other's.

What's more, accurate health information helps children understand the complexities of the world around them. Today's children face a different world than their parents and grandparents did at the same age. Their lives are often more scheduled (and sometimes more pressured); their leisure time is filled with television, technological gadgets, and video games. Adolescents of both sexes seem to be maturing earlier than previous generations. Girls are bombarded with exposure to provocative fashions and the media's obsession with superstars (whose personal choices are often less than healthy!). Boys, meanwhile, are exposed to confusing messages about sex, violence, and decision-making. Both sexes face a social world where drugs are readily available. Kids today—like the rest of us—need clearly presented, accurate health information more than ever.

Meanwhile, it often seems as though we are confronted with health information everywhere we turn: on the news, on the Internet, in TV ads, and from our friends and relatives. Too often we receive conflicting messages. Should we eat butter—or margarine? Are eggs unhealthy? Are certain medications safe or not? The answers to these and other questions are often confusing. It is difficult to know what sources to trust and how to find the best information.

This encyclopedia will help you overcome this dilemma. It presents a collection of accurate and up-to-date information that parents and children can trust. It's arranged in an easy-to-access alphabetical format that provides an overview of all areas of health and wellness. The 10 volumes cover a wealth of information, including human anatomy and physiology, diseases and disorders, treatments and cures, and prevention and diagnosis. The books address the concerns of both young children and adults, as well as today's teens and tweens, with topics such as abstinence and pregnancy, drug addiction and smoking, cancer and STDs, and much more. The "Ask the Doctor" sections pose questions that are on the minds of many kids today—questions kids may be afraid to ask out loud. The information provided is current, factual, and presented in a straightforward manner. The artwork is carefully selected to illustrate the text and bring alive topics that might otherwise be hard to grasp.

Keep in mind that these books should never be used in place of consulting a health practitioner. They're intended merely to give you a clear overview of the topics, facilitating your communication with your health-care provider. With that proviso, it is my hope that these volumes will contribute to your understanding of health and wellness, and that they will help you and your families cope with the many health challenges that confront us all.

I encourage you to use these books as one building block in your family's well-being. May you enjoy them in good health!

—Dr. Elise Berlan

Immune System

IMMUNE SYSTEM

The immune system protects the body from **pathogens** and abnormalities that could cause illness. It also "cleans" the body by removing dead or damaged tissue. The human immune system is an incredibly complex network of organs, tissues, **cells**, and other components that all work together, providing multiple layers of protection. In humans, the immune system offers three basic forms of protection: physical barriers, the innate immune system, and the adaptive immune system.

Physical Barriers

The immune system's physical barriers are all the things designed to keep unwanted invaders out of the body. The **skin** is the largest and most obvious barrier. It protects everything inside the body. When pathogens like **viruses** and **bacteria** penetrate this barrier, it is usually through a cut or other opening in the skin. Some harmful substances, like certain chemicals, can also be absorbed through the skin. The small hairs lining the **nose** are another type of barrier. They work in concert with **mucus** to filter out particles and pathogens of the air that is inhaled.

Endothelial cells are another type of barrier. They are the cells that line the **blood vessels**' inner walls.

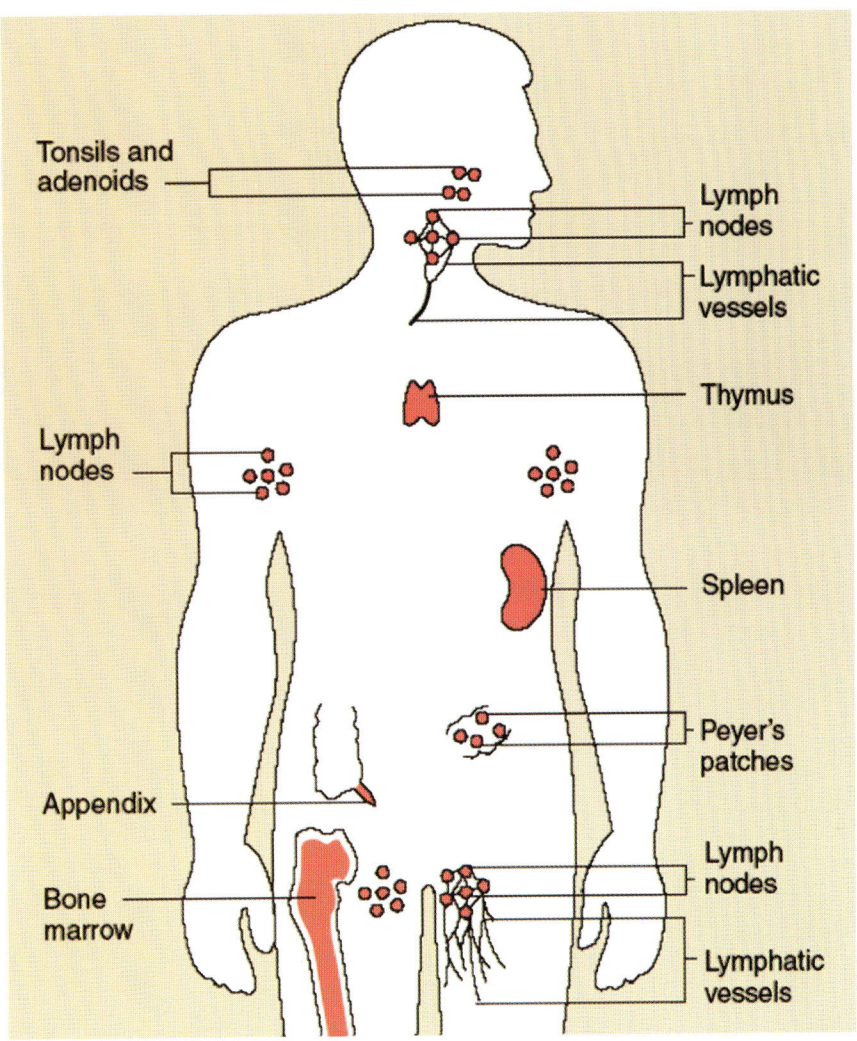

The immune system has many parts, all working together to protect the body against disease and infection.

Immune System

Their major function is to help blood flow through the vessels, but they also perform a barrier function, especially in the blood vessels of the **brain**. In the brain, there are many more endothelial cells in the blood vessels. They are packed tightly together to form something called the blood-brain barrier. These tightly packed cells make it much harder for harmful substances to escape the blood stream and get into the brain. The blood-brain barrier is another important part of the immune system's physical barrier system.

Innate Immune Response

If a pathogen manages to get past the initial barriers, it will meet the body's innate immune system. This is a nonspecific immune response, meaning the response is the same regardless of the type of pathogen. The innate immune system creates chemical reactions that cause inflammation and call immune cells to the site of **infection**. As the area becomes inflamed, blood and certain types of chemicals flood to the site, causing heat, redness, and swelling. The purpose of inflammation is to make it harder for the pathogen to spread and to attract white blood cells that kill infective agents. The innate immune system is triggered when pathogens like viruses and bacteria enter the body. But substances called allergens—things like pollen, mold spores, dust, animal dander, and other substances that may cause an allergic reaction—can

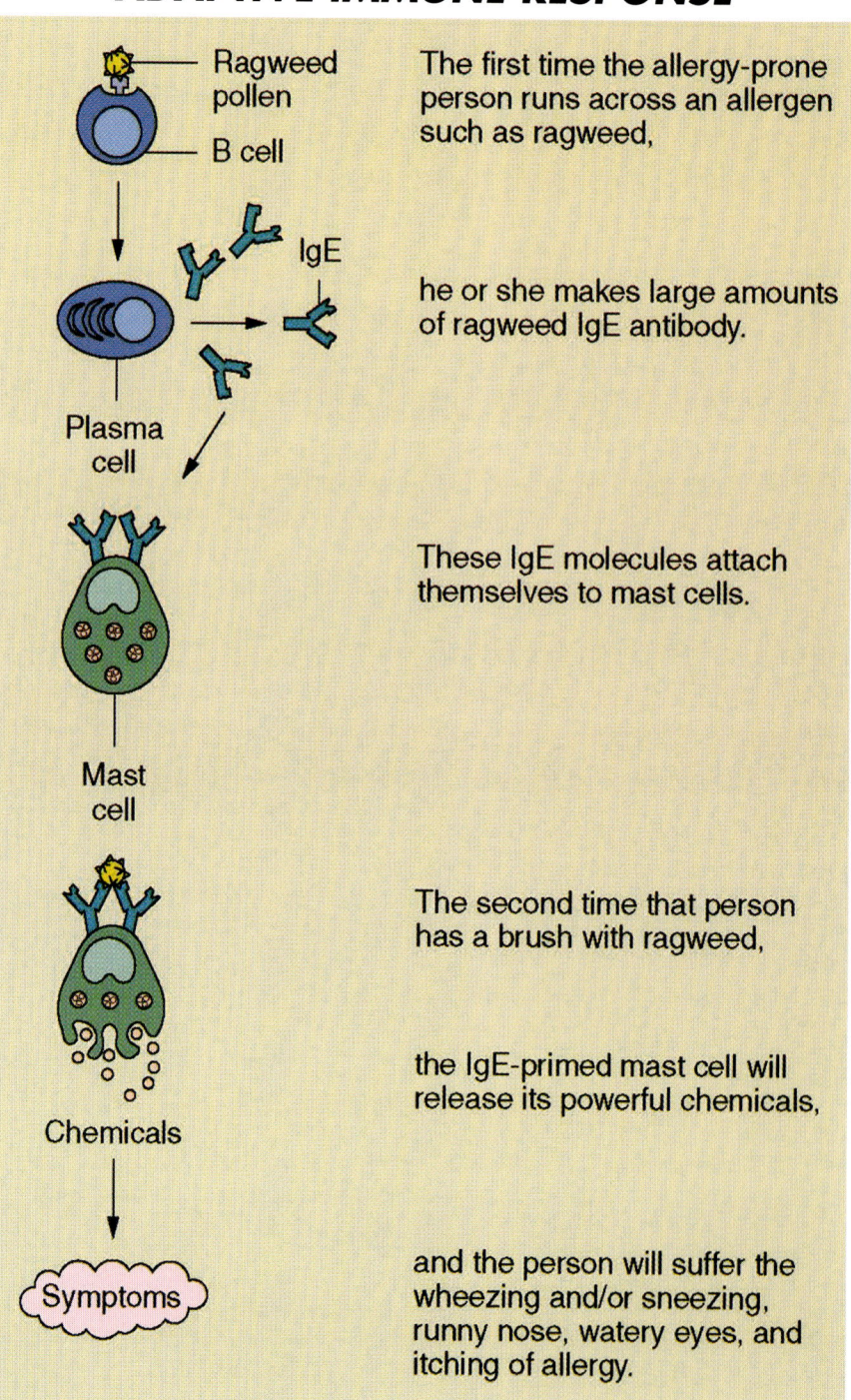

ADAPTIVE IMMUNE RESPONSE

The first time the allergy-prone person runs across an allergen such as ragweed,

he or she makes large amounts of ragweed IgE antibody.

These IgE molecules attach themselves to mast cells.

The second time that person has a brush with ragweed,

the IgE-primed mast cell will release its powerful chemicals,

and the person will suffer the wheezing and/or sneezing, runny nose, watery eyes, and itching of allergy.

also trigger it. Allergic reactions are reactions of the innate immune system.

Adaptive Immune Response

For some body invaders, the innate immune response will be enough to destroy the pathogen and prevent infection. If the infection is large enough, however, the innate immune system will activate the adaptive (or specific) immune system. Unlike the innate immune system, which treats all invaders the same way, the adaptive immune system distinguishes between different pathogens, tailors an immune response specific to that pathogen, and "remembers" the pathogen so it can be eliminated quicker and more efficiently in the event of future exposure. The ability of the adaptive immune system to remember specific pathogens is called "immunological memory." It is an extremely important immune function that only exists in vertebrates. In the case of the adaptive immune system, the old phrase, "What doesn't kill you makes you stronger," holds true. Every infection the organism survives leads to a "strengthening" of the immune system through the creation of specific cells that will be able to quickly recognize and fight off that infection in the future.

Autoimmune Disorders

Autoimmune disorders are conditions in which a person's immune system treats her own cells and tissues as foreign entities and attacks them. A very low level of autoimmunity is probably always present in the body, and is even thought to be beneficial, specifically in killing precancerous and cancerous cells before they can multiply and harm the body. It is only when autoimmunity becomes

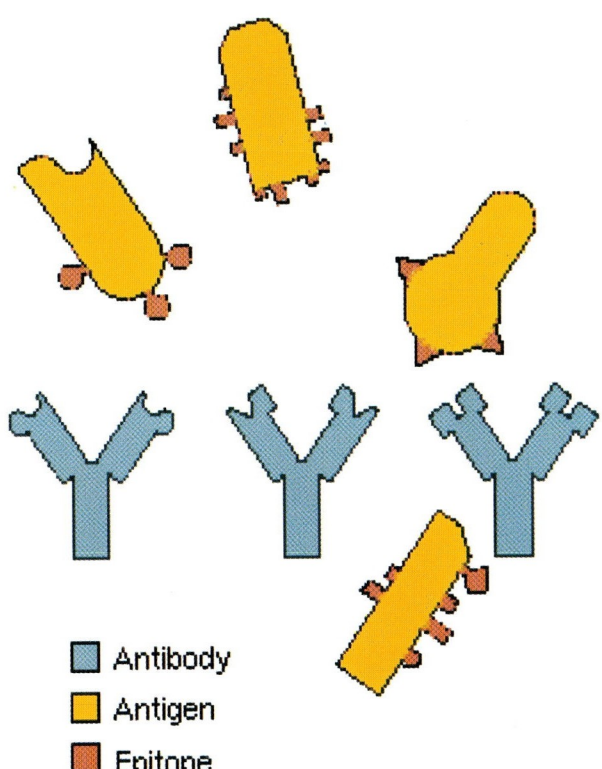

Antibodies are blood proteins that allow the immune system to identify and neutralize germs. Antigens are another type of molecule, also part of the immune system. Epitopes are "tags" on molecules to which antibodies can bind.

overactive that it is considered a disorder and results in adverse effects.

There are many different autoimmune disorders, and they can affect different parts and systems of the body. Some are relatively benign, while others are extremely dangerous. An example of a relatively benign autoimmune disorder is vitiligo. In this condition, the immune system attacks the body's pigment cells, causing often-permanent white patches on the skin and hair. Vitiligo causes changes in a person's appearance, but it is not believed to have other adverse health effects. In that sense, it is largely a cosmetic condition. However, severe vitiligo can still be extremely distressing to the individual experiencing it, especially for people who have

Immune System

ASK THE DOCTOR

My mom said she has an autoimmune disorder. Does that mean she has AIDS?

A: No. An autoimmune disorder is different from AIDS, which stands for acquired immunodeficiency syndrome. A specific virus called HIV (or human immunodeficiency virus) causes this syndrome. HIV attacks a person's immune system, causing immunodeficiency, which makes the person susceptible to certain infections and cancers. A virus does not directly cause an autoimmune disorder. It is a malfunctioning of the immune system that makes the immune system attack the person's body. In a way, we can think of immunodeficiency as an underactive immune system, and an autoimmune disorder as an overactive immune system.

"vitiligo spots" on the face or have darker skin, making the white patches extremely noticeable. In certain cases, individuals with severe vitiligo may feel disfigured and suffer additional symptoms, like increased stress and decreased social interactions, due to their feelings about their appearance. These complications, however, are caused by a psychological reaction to the condition, rather than by the physical condition itself.

An example of a more physically damaging and dangerous autoimmune disorder is systemic lupus erythematosus, often called simply SLE or lupus. In this condition, the autoimmune response is highly overactive and wages an attack on the body's cells and tissues. Certain parts of the body are frequently attacked by lupus. The skin is often attacked, causing thick, scaly, red patches on the body and/or a butterfly-shaped **rash** on the face. The **joints** are also commonly attacked, causing soreness, pain, and stiffness. Major organs, such as the **lungs**, **heart**, **liver**, and **kidneys**, are also often affected, which can cause severe complications, disability, and sometimes even death. With advances in medical treatment, however, lupus is no longer as frequently fatal as it once was.

Rheumatoid arthritis (RA), in which tissues of the joints are attacked, is yet another example of a severe and debilitating autoimmune disorder. It is a progressive disease, meaning it gets worse as time goes on. Individuals with RA may have systems in as little as one joint or, more

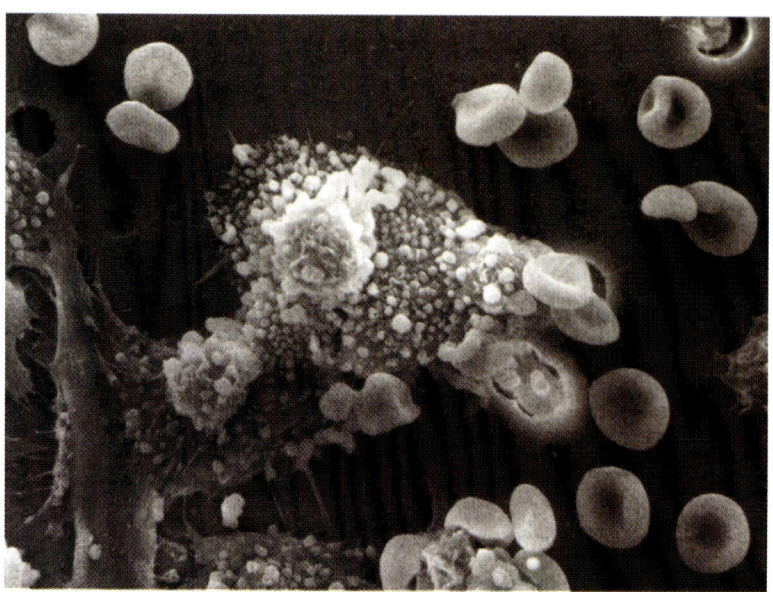

This magnified image shows the immune system's cells combating cancer cells. Patrolling cells provide continuous body-wide surveillance, catching and eliminating cells if they begin to turn cancerous. Tumors develop when this immune surveillance breaks down or is overwhelmed.

14

Immune System

> **DID YOU KNOW?**
>
> *When a foreign particle (a flu virus, for instance) invades your body, it has different proteins than the ones normally found in your body. If an immune cell happens to bump into and recognize the virus, it immediately knows to destroy that cell. Special "warrior cells" (called T cells) in your blood become programmed to find and destroy all cells displaying the foreign proteins. Before long, the original T cells will have produced a tiny army of cells ready to fight off the infection. When a T cell makes contact with a flu-infected cell, it injects a protein that pokes holes in the cell and very quickly destroys it.*

commonly, in many joints. As the disease condition progresses and worsens, the number of joints affected usually increases. Symptoms are often worse in the morning, with greater pain and stiffness. The pain and stiffness can make movement difficult, but most people with RA find that using and exercising the affected area reduces the pain and stiffness. This becomes more difficult over time, however, as the condition leads to permanent damage and destruction of joint tissues, resulting in decreased mobility and sometimes, especially in the case of the fingers, in gradual deformation of the affected area.

Vitiligo, lupus, and rheumatoid arthritis are just three examples of autoimmune disorders, but there are many others. Autoimmune disorders can be unpredictable, flaring up or going into remission, sometimes with no apparent cause. Many are chronic, meaning they are always present or have the potential to recur. Chronic autoimmune disorders may be treated, but are never fully cured. Things like hormonal changes, **stress**, and illness may trigger flare-ups of certain autoimmune conditions. Autoimmune disorders are generally treated with medications. Corticosteroids, which are hormones that perform a number of functions in the body, are often used to reduce inflammation. Immunosuppressants, which inhibit the immune system resulting in decreased immune responses and therefore decreased autoimmune responses, may also be used.

Immunodeficiency

Immunodeficiency is when an abnormally weak immune system leads to an inability to properly fight disease and infection. There are different types of immunodeficiency, and immunodeficiency conditions can be **congenital**, meaning present from **birth**, or acquired, meaning they develop later in life. If a person's immunodeficiency is the result of a condition present since birth, it is called primary immunodeficiency. Primary forms of immunodeficiency are often inherited; they have a **genetic** component and run in families. Acquired forms of immunodeficiency, also called secondary immunodeficiency, are far more common than primary forms. Things like **malnutrition**, certain medications, and diseases can cause acquired immunodeficiency. Human immunodeficiency virus (**HIV**) causes immunodeficiency by attacking the immune system and destroying cells responsible for fighting disease.

Immune System

Immunodeficiency can also be purposefully induced through suppression of the immune system. This is usually done for a medical purpose. For example, a person receiving an organ or tissue transplant must have his immune system suppressed so that his body will not attack and reject the transplant. People with immunodeficiency, whether it is primary, secondary, or purposefully induced, are at an increased risk of developing illnesses and infections, and those illnesses and infections can be far more severe and dangerous than in individuals with normally functioning immune systems.

For more information, visit the National Institute of Allergy and Infectious Disease:
www.niaid.nih.gov/final/immun/immun.htm

IMMUNIZATION

Immunization, also called **vaccination**, gives an individual a small dose of pathogenic material or some other substance to induce an immune response that will lead to long-term immunity to a certain disease. Immunization usually involves injection of a vaccine with a needle, but there are also some oral vaccines and other forms of immunization.

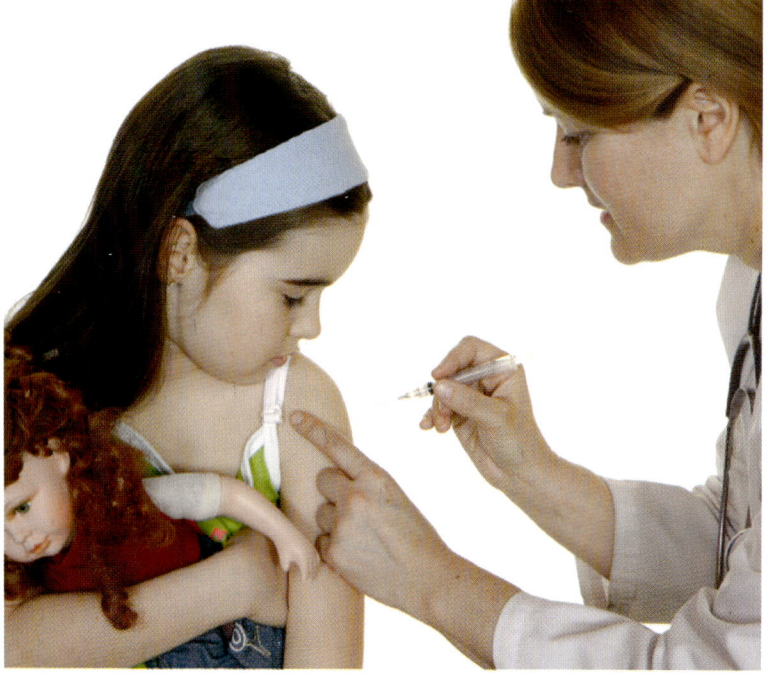

ASK THE DOCTOR
I have a friend who says vaccines are dangerous. Is this true?

A: Millions of people's lives are saved every year by immunization. Throughout the history of immunization, there have been occasional cases of people having adverse reactions to vaccines, of vaccines being tainted with harmful substances, of people getting sick from the vaccine itself, of vaccines being inadequately tested before entering the market and then having to be withdrawn, and other problems. But all of these problems pale in comparison to the vast benefits of immunization. The diseases we immunize against have the potential to kill or cause lifelong disability. Today, hundreds of millions of people owe their lives or unimpaired health to vaccination, and practically every person on earth has benefited from immunization in some way.

The immune system recognizes the dead or harmless germs in a vaccine as foreign substances, destroys them, and then "remembers" them. When the dangerous version of the germ comes along, the body recognizes it and destroys it.

Recommended Immunization Schedule for Persons Aged 0–6 Years—UNITED STATES • 2008

From the Department for Health and Human Services and the Centers for Disease Control and Prevention

Vaccine ▼ Age ▶	Birth	1 month	2 months	4 months	6 months	12 months	15 months	18 months	19–23 months	2–3 years	4–6 years
Hepatitis B	HepB	HepB			HepB						
Rotavirus			Rota	Rota	Rota						
Diphtheria, Tetanus, Pertussis			DTaP	DTaP	DTaP		DTaP				DTaP
Haemophilus influenzae type b			Hib	Hib	Hib'	Hib					
Pneumococcal			PCV	PCV	PCV	PCV				PPV	
Inactivated Poliovirus			IPV	IPV	IPV						IPV
Influenza					Influenza (Yearly)						
Measles, Mumps, Rubella						MMR					MMR
Varicella						Varicella					Varicella
Hepatitis A						HepA (2 doses)				HepA Series	
Meningococcal											MCV4

Range of recommended ages

Certain high-risk groups

Immunizations are waging war on once-common illnesses, such as rubella, polio, and typhoid. Thanks to parents seeing that their children follow the immunization schedule above, these diseases are nowhere near as common as they were just a hundred years ago.

Immunization is a way of exposing people to dangerous diseases in small, controlled, low-risk doses. This exposure triggers the body to produce the antibodies necessary for recognizing and fighting the infection. Then, when the person comes in contact with the full-strength disease, she will already have immunity and won't get sick. Immunization has greatly reduced people's risk of death or disability from many diseases.

In some countries, immunization has virtually wiped out certain diseases. **Smallpox** is the only disease, however, that is believed to have been completely eradicated by immunization. A century ago, smallpox was a worldwide killer of millions of people each year. When a vaccine was developed, however, everything changed. After many decades of concerted effort to vaccinate the world population, smallpox was finally declared extinct by the World Health Organization (WHO) in 1979. Today, children no longer get immunized against smallpox because the disease is believed to no longer exist in nature.

Not all immunization campaigns, however, have been as successful as that against smallpox. Many diseases are still major killers with no way to currently immunize against them. Malaria is an example of one such disease. Research is currently underway to develop a vaccine for malaria.

For more information visit the Centers for Disease Control and Prevention at: www.cdc.gov/vaccines

IMPOTENCE

Impotence, also called erectile dysfunction, is the inability of a male to achieve or

17

Impotence

maintain **erection**. Erectile dysfunction (ED) is more common in men over age 65, but it can occur at any age. In fact, it is normal for most men to experience an occasional episode of ED. The cause of erectile dysfunction can be either psychological or physical. Physical causes of ED include nerve damage, certain medications, cardiovascular disorders, spinal cord injuries, hormonal disorders, and substance abuse. The most common psychological problems include stress, anxiety, and fatigue. Negative feelings towards a sexual partner, such as resentment, hostility or disinterest can also be a factor.

Though an occasional occurrence of impotence is normal, when ED begins to be a persistent problem, it can interfere with a man's sexual life as well as his self-image. Erectile dysfunction may be a difficult topic for a man to discuss, but a visit to his doctor can diagnose underlying causes and offer several treatment options.

For more information visit the Mayo Clinic at: www.mayoclinic.com/health/erectile-dysfunction/DS00162/DSECTION=1

INCONTINENCE

Incontinence is impairment in one's ability to retain urine or feces until they can be consciously expelled. The inability to control urination is called urinary incontinence. The inability to control feces is called fecal incontinence.

Fecal Incontinence

Fecal incontinence is the inability to effectively control the bowels, leading to unintentional loss of fecal matter. Fecal incontinence can have a number of causes. Some forms of fecal incontinence may be temporary and clear on their own when the underlying cause resolves itself. Examples of this are incontinence caused by severe **diarrhea** and by certain medications. Other forms of fecal incontinence are more long-lasting and require treatment if there is to be any improvement in the condition. An example of this is incontinence caused by **muscle** or **nerve** damage.

The most common cause of fecal incontinence (that is not due to temporary illness or medication) is damage to the internal sphincter, the external sphincter, or both. These sphincters are ring-shaped muscles, located at the end of the rectum near the anus, that assist in holding fecal matter inside the body until it is ready to be expelled. The most common cause of damage to these muscles in women is childbirth, especially episiotomy (the cutting of the perineum, which is located between the **vagina** and the **anus**). Certain types of surgery may also damage the sphincter muscles in both men and women. In some cases of fecal incontinence due to malfunctioning sphincter muscles, the muscles themselves may be undamaged, but the nerves that control them are impaired. Again, this may be due to childbirth, surgery, or other causes.

Treatment options for fecal incontinence include medications, exercises to help strengthen weak or damaged muscles (these may be especially necessary and helpful during recovery from surgery or childbirth), surgery, changes in diet, and implantation of a device that sends electrical signals to nerves involved in stool retention and expulsion. Diapers that contain unintentional stool loss are also a common part of treatment, and many patients may need a combination of treatments to achieve the best possible results.

Urinary Incontinence

A number of things can cause urinary incontinence. One of the most common forms of incontinence in both men and women is stress incontinence. This is when small amounts of urine are squeezed from the body when a person does something that increases abdominal pressure. Many activities and movements, like **coughing**, **sneezing**, laughing, and exercising, increase abdominal pressure (and pressure on the **bladder**). In stress incontinence, the muscles in the pelvic floor responsible for holding urine in the bladder aren't strong enough or don't respond quickly enough to hold in urine when pressure is quickly increased. Some of the most common causes of stress incontinence are weakening of the pelvic floor muscles during **pregnancy** and childbirth in women, or as a complication following **prostate**-removal surgery in men.

Another form of urinary incontinence is hypertonic (or urge) incontinence. Some other common names for this condition are overactive or spastic bladder. In this condition, the person feels a sudden need to urinate and then releases urine. There are two primary causes of urge incontinence: having an infection of the bladder, or a disease or injury affecting the nerves and/or muscles

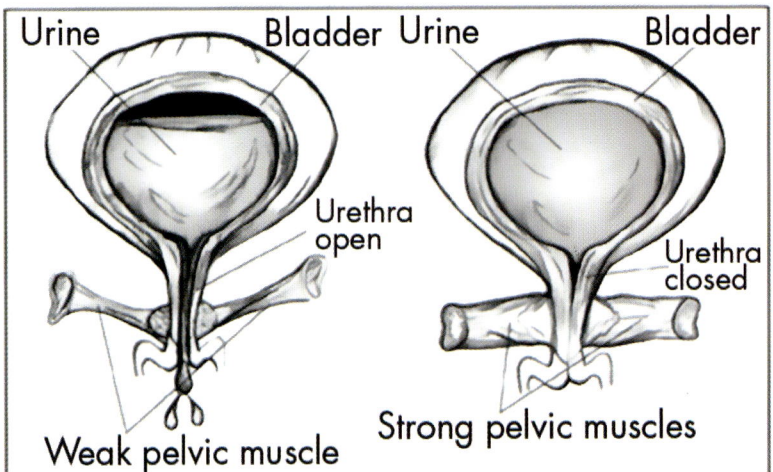

The pressure from a full bladder may be too much for weak muscles to contain; when this happens, drops of urine may escape. Strengthening pelvic muscles through exercise can help prevent this.

ASK THE DOCTOR

My friends say that when you get pregnant, sometimes you wet your pants. Is this true?

A: Incontinence is, unfortunately, a common experience in pregnancy, especially in the final weeks when the baby is very large and the uterus is pressing heavily on the bladder. A significant number of women will experience stress incontinence at this stage in pregnancy. Some women also find that, when they have to urinate, they have trouble holding it until they reach a toilet. Luckily, this type of incontinence usually resolves after the baby is born and pressure on the bladder is relieved. But incontinence can also be a problem after pregnancy due to weakening of muscles or damage suffered during the birth process. Furthermore, incontinence can occur years or decades later because of changes that occurred in the body during pregnancy and childbirth. A lot of people are embarrassed by incontinence, and therefore try to deny, hide, or manage the problem themselves instead of speaking with a doctor. This is a mistake. Many forms of incontinency are quite treatable. Sometimes just doing some simple exercises is enough to solve the problem.

Incontinence

responsible for urinary control. Diseases that can cause urge incontinence include *multiple sclerosis* and *Parkinson's disease*. *Stroke* and injuries that cause nerve damage and *paralysis* can also result in urge incontinence.

There is also a type of incontinence called overflow incontinence, where the bladder seems to always be full and continuously leaking, or urine continues to dribble for a long time after conscious urination. This type of incontinence can have different causes, including something pinching or obstructing the urethra (the tube that transports urine), weak bladder muscles, or neurological damage. A type of incontinence called functional incontinence can also occur when a person has some type of impairment that makes him unable to get to the toilet or realize that they need to use the toilet in time to use it. This may happen because of diseases, like *Alzheimer's* disease, that affect mental functioning, or because of impaired mobility, especially due to advanced age.

There are treatments available for incontinence, including medications and surgeries. The type of treatment and the level of success that can be expected from it, however, depend largely on the underlying cause of the incontinence.

For more information visit the National Association for Continence at: www.nafc.org/about_incontinence/what_incontinence.htm

INDIGESTION

Indigestion, often called "upset stomach," is disruption of the digestive tract that can result in pain, bloating, *heartburn*, belching, and other symptoms. Some causes of indigestion include food *allergies* or sensitivities, *stress*, or bacterial levels in food.

Occasional indigestion is usually nothing to worry about, but if indigestion is persistent it may be caused by a more serious underlying condition.

> Some digestive conditions that may cause indigestion include:
>
> - heartburn, or acid reflux, which occurs when stomach acid backs up into the esophagus
> - peptic ulcers—open sores on the stomach lining
> - gastritis—inflammation of the stomach lining
> - gallstones—solid deposits of cholesterol or calcium salts that form in the gallbladder
> - stomach cancer
>
> Consult your doctor if you experience symptoms such as weight loss; vomiting; change in stools; shortness of breath; or pain in the jaw, neck, or arm.

For most people, the right lifestyle choices can help prevent episodes of indigestion. Avoiding overindulgence in fatty or spicy foods, eating slowly or limiting intake of alcoholic beverages can prevent many cases of upset stomach. Good stress management and regular *exercise* are also healthy choices that can help you avoid indigestion.

For more information, visit the National Digestive Diseases Information Clearinghouse: digestive.niddk.nih.gov/ddiseases/pubs/indigestion

INFECTION AND INFECTIOUS DISEASES

Infection is when a *pathogen* enters the body and begins to reproduce and flourish,

Infection & Infectious Diseases

establishing a colony. **Bacteria** and **viruses** are the most common causes of infection, but other organisms or substances, such as **parasites**, fungi, or prions can also cause illness.

Bacteria, viruses, and other infectious agents are constantly present in and entering the human body, but they are normally destroyed by the **immune system** before they can reproduce (or replicate), establish a colony, and cause damage to the body. When a bacteria or virus manages to establish itself and multiply, the person is said to have an infection. Not all bacteria and viruses, however, are dangerous to humans. Many types of bacteria, for example, are part of the body's natural flora and are even beneficial to the body's functioning.

A pathogen that can colonize on or inside a person's body—meaning the bacteria, virus, or other invader can establish a strong, reproducing population—is said to be "infective"; it is capable of infecting. Not all infective agents will cause damage or disease

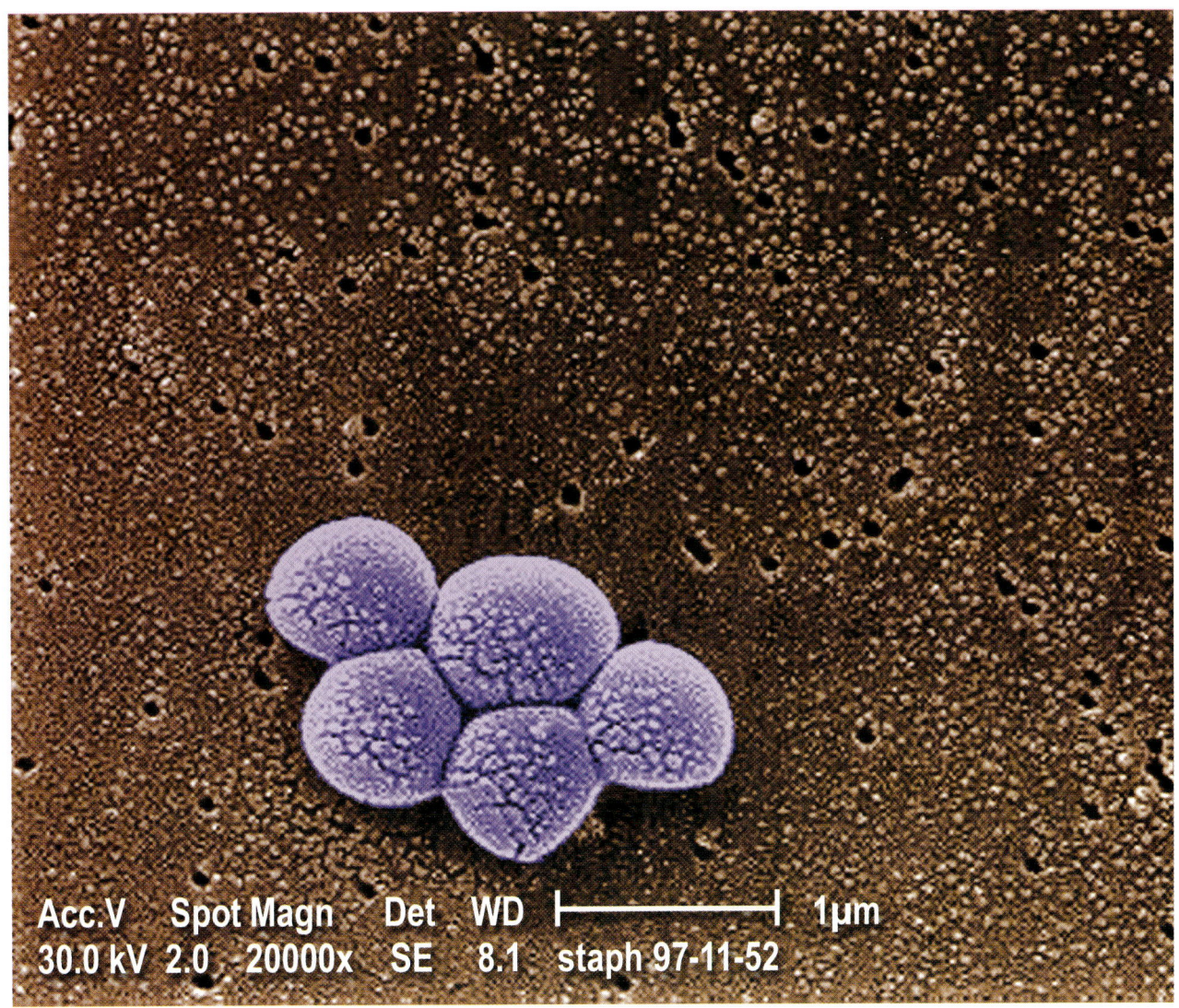

This magnified image shows staph cells—otherwise known as *Staphylococcus aureus*, an extremely common form of bacteria. Most of us have some living on our skin all the time, but when this bacteria enters the body, usually through a break in the skin, it can cause infection anywhere.

Infection & Infectious Diseases

to the infected person. Sometimes a person can have a minor infection and not know it at all. The body's immune system will usually fight off the infection. At other times, however, an infection adversely affects the body and makes the person ill. When this happens, the person is experiencing "disease." If the infective agent and resulting disease can be spread to other people, the person is said to have an "infectious disease."

Primary Pathogens

There are many different kinds of infectious diseases in the world. Infectious diseases are usually categorized in one of two ways. The most common are "primary" pathogens (or infections). Primary pathogens are those capable of overwhelming healthy immune systems, causing disease in otherwise healthy individuals. Examples of primary pathogens are the **influenza** virus, which causes respiratory infection and other symptoms commonly referred to as "flu"; **tuberculosis** (TB), a deadly lung infection caused by a type of bacteria called mycobacteria; and **malaria**, a blood infection caused by a very tiny parasite. These, of course, are only a few examples of primary pathogens.

Opportunistic Pathogens

Opportunistic pathogens are those that are fought off by healthy immune systems and will not cause disease in healthy people. However, they are called "opportunistic" because, when a person has a weakened or compromised immune system (such as a person whose immune system has been suppressed for organ transplant or a person who has **AIDS**), the pathogen takes the opportunity to invade and colonize. When a person develops a disease from an opportunistic infection, it is almost always a sign that there is an underlying problem with that person's immune system. Some examples of opportunistic pathogens include *Candida albicans*, a type of fungus that is harmlessly present in most people, but causes oral and genital infections in immune-compromised individuals; *Human herpesvirus 8*, which causes bruise-like lesions and tumors called Kaposi's sarcoma, usually in people with **HIV/AIDS**; and *Toxoplasma gondii*, a parasitic infection that causes toxoplasmosis, which is generally not dangerous but can be fatal to the human fetus or to people with compromised immune systems.

Infectious Disease Transmission

A defining feature of infectious diseases is that they can be spread from the host (the infected individual), or from some other source, to other people. This is true for both primary and opportunistic pathogens. Infectious diseases can be spread in a number of different ways depending on the type of pathogen. The way a disease spreads is called its "mode of transmission."

WASH YOUR HANDS!

Hands spread an estimated 80% of common infectious diseases. The best way to prevent this? Always wash your hands with soap and water after you use the bathroom, before and after handling food, after coughing or sneezing, after contact with animals, and after sharing a toy or other item.

Airborne Transmission

Airborne transmission can occur when a pathogen, like a virus, is able to survive in the air for long periods of time, where it

Infection & Infectious Diseases

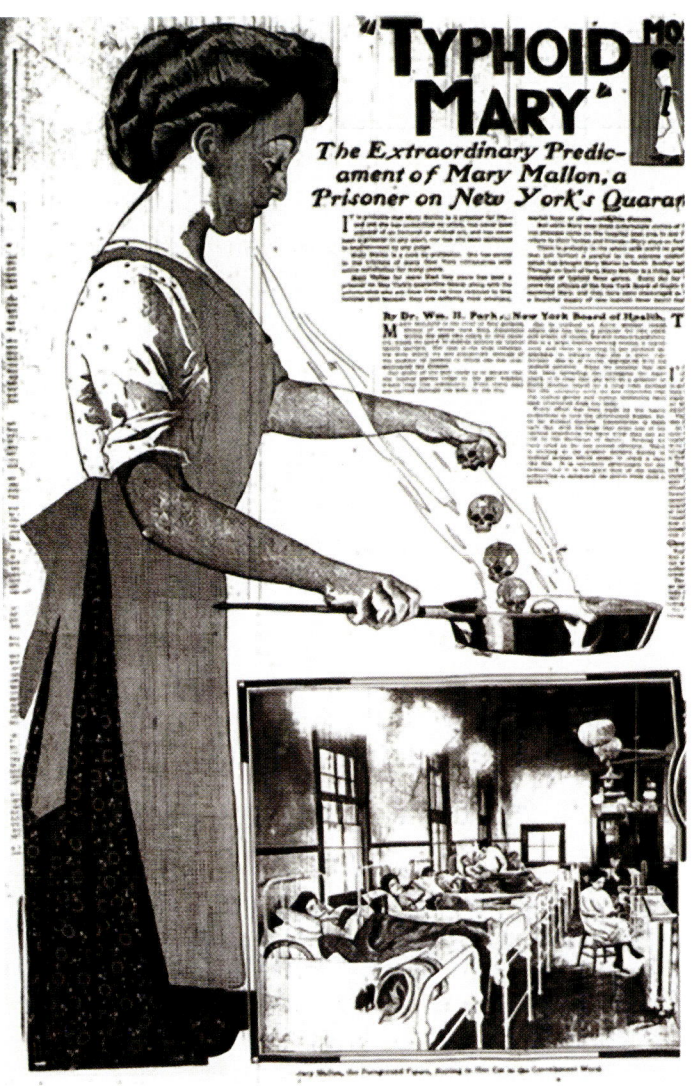

Typhoid fever is a deadly disease caused by *Salmonella typhi*, a bacillus found in human urine and feces. At the beginning of the 20th century, "Typhoid Mary," an immigrant woman named Mary Mallon, was called "the most dangerous woman in America" because she spread typhoid to as many as eight households. When a doctor became suspicious and tracked her down, Mary admitted that she rarely washed her hands while cooking. Authorities confined her to a cottage in the Bronx, where she lived and ate alone for four years. Finally, when she promised to become a laundress and never return to cooking, Mary was released. She changed her name to Mary Brown and got a job as a cook. For the next five years, she went through a series of kitchens, spreading illness and death, until the police found her. This time she was quarantined for life. Exactly how many people she infected or killed will never be known.

can then be inhaled or otherwise acquired by people moving through/using that air. Airborne transmission is not a particularly common mode of transmission, since there are relatively few pathogens that can survive in the air long enough to be transmitted from person to person. Infectious agents that are capable of airborne transmission can be extremely dangerous because they can pass nearly uninhibited from person to person.

Direct Physical Contact

Sometimes a new host must come in direct physical contact with the infected person in order for a pathogen to spread. Ringworm, a rash caused by a fungus, is an example of a pathogen that passes through direct physical contact (although it can also be spread through indirect contact). For some pathogens, like ringworm, casual physical contact, like shaking hands or brushing against someone's skin, can be enough to transmit the pathogen. For many infectious diseases, however, the physical contact needs to be more involved. Sexual transmission is perhaps the most common way that diseases are spread through direct physical contact.

Droplet Transmission

Droplet transmission is another of the most common ways infectious diseases are transmitted from one person to another. This is particularly true for illnesses like the **common cold** and **flu** that affect the **respiratory system**. In droplet transmission, droplets of respiratory fluid (such as **mucus** from the **nose**) are passed from one person to another. The virus or other infectious agent is suspended in this fluid. The respiratory droplet acts like a little ecosystem or biosphere where the pathogen can live until it is spread to a new host. The respiratory droplets, also called aerosols, are usually spread when an infected person coughs or sneezes onto another person. The droplets can also be spread (by coughing, sneezing, touching, etc.) onto the hands and then transmitted to other people or objects. Droplet transmission can also occur by sharing things like glasses and eating utensils.

Fecal-Oral Transmission

Fecal-oral spread is how most gastrointestinal illnesses are transmitted. Fecal-oral spread is when another individual ingests fecal matter from a germ host. This may happen when, for example, someone uses the bathroom and gets microscopic amounts of fecal matter on his hands, doesn't wash his hands, and then consumes food. It also commonly occurs when water or food supplies become contaminated by, for example, a breakdown in water filtration systems, run-off from farms that carries fecal matter from animals into water supplies, or when fecal matter contaminates meat during butchering and processing.

Horizontal Transmission

Horizontal transmission is a term used to describe how a disease moves through a population. It is when disease moves from any individual to any other individual through airborne transmission, droplet transmission, direct contact, fecal-oral transmission, indirect contact, sexual transmission, or vector-borne transmission.

Indirect Contact

Some pathogens can be spread through indirect contact. Unlike direct contact transmission, a person does not have to come into actual physical contact with an infected person to acquire the infectious agent. The infectious agent may be left behind on surfaces or objects that an infected person has used, or it may contaminate soil, food, or other communal resources. Anyone who comes in contact with the contamination may then also acquire the infectious agent.

Sexual Transmission

Many infections are spread through sexual contact. They are usually called sexually transmitted infections (STIs). The pathogens that cause these infections are present in blood, semen, and vaginal fluid. During unprotected sexual contact, body fluids are exchanged, leading to a very high risk of an infected person passing an STI on to the person they have had sexual contact with. Some sexually transmitted infections, such as the herpes simplex virus and the human

DID YOU KNOW?

Most people have heard the term STD, which stands for sexually transmitted diseases. Increasingly, the term STI, or sexually transmitted infections, is being used because infection has a broader ranger of meaning than disease. Infection refers to the first step, when a pathogen enters the body and begins multiplying. Disease is the result of an infection—cells are damaged, and the signs and symptoms of an illness appear.

Infection & Infectious Diseases

ASK THE DOCTOR

If a woman has HIV and has a baby, will the baby also have HIV?

A: Not necessarily. In fact, today if medications are used and proper procedures are followed during childbirth and in the postpartum period, the vast majority of babies with HIV-positive mothers can actually be born HIV free. This is because, from the very beginning, the developing fetus has a different blood supply from its mother. While in the womb, the fetus is nourished by nutrients filtering out of the mother's blood stream and into the placenta. There, nutrients are picked up by an independent blood supply that is flowing through the fetus and placenta. The placenta acts as a type of barrier or gatekeeper. It allows nutrients to be transferred from the mother to the fetus, but without blood being shared. The HIV virus is in the mother's blood, but it can't pass through the placental barrier. The greatest risk for transmission from mother to child, then, occurs during the birth process, when fluids from the mother's body might enter the child's body. Proper treatment during pregnancy, precautions and medications during the birth process, and antiviral treatment of the newborn reduce the odds of vertical HIV transmission to about 2 to 3 in every 100 births.

papilloma virus, may be spread by direct skin-to-skin contact as well. Other examples of sexually transmitted infections include chlamydia, HIV, and gonorrhea. Condom use does prevent the transmission of many sexually transmitted infections.

Vector-Borne Transmission

Vector-borne transmission occurs when a pathogen is spread from person to person via another carrier, often an insect or animal. Vectors are third parties that allow pathogens to spread from individual to individual without those individuals ever actually coming into contact with each other. The vector can house the pathogen without being harmed by it. Vectors in which the pathogen multiplies and reproduces are called "biological" vectors. Vectors that simply transport the pathogen from one place to another, but don't play any role in its life cycle, are called "mechanical" vectors.

Mosquitoes are common vectors, particularly for the parasite that causes malaria. When the mosquito bites and sucks the blood of a person with malaria, it ingests the tiny parasite. The next time it bites a person, it may spread the parasite on. Some species of mosquitoes are also vectors for West Nile virus. Ticks are vectors for a number of diseases (for example, **Lyme disease**), while fleas are vectors for several other illnesses, including bubonic plague.

Vertical Transmission

Vertical transmission is when a disease moves from parent to offspring. This is in contrast to horizontal transmission, in which a disease moves through a population regardless of the individuals' relationships to each other. In vertical transmission, a disease moves from the parent to the child during gestation, birth, or breastfeeding. A baby contracting HIV during the birth process from its HIV-positive mother would be an example of vertical transmission.

For more information visit the National Center for Infectious Diseases at: www.cdc.gov/ncidod

INFECTIOUS MONO-NUCLEOSIS

Infectious mononucleosis, commonly called "mono" or "the kissing disease," is an illness that affects the immune system causing **flu**-like symptoms and **fatigue**. The fatigue is extreme in some people and is a defining symptom of the illness.

The **virus** that causes mononucleosis is *Human herpesvirus 4* (HHV-4), also known as Epstein-Barr virus (EBV). Many people become infected with this virus but never develop any symptoms or illness. In other

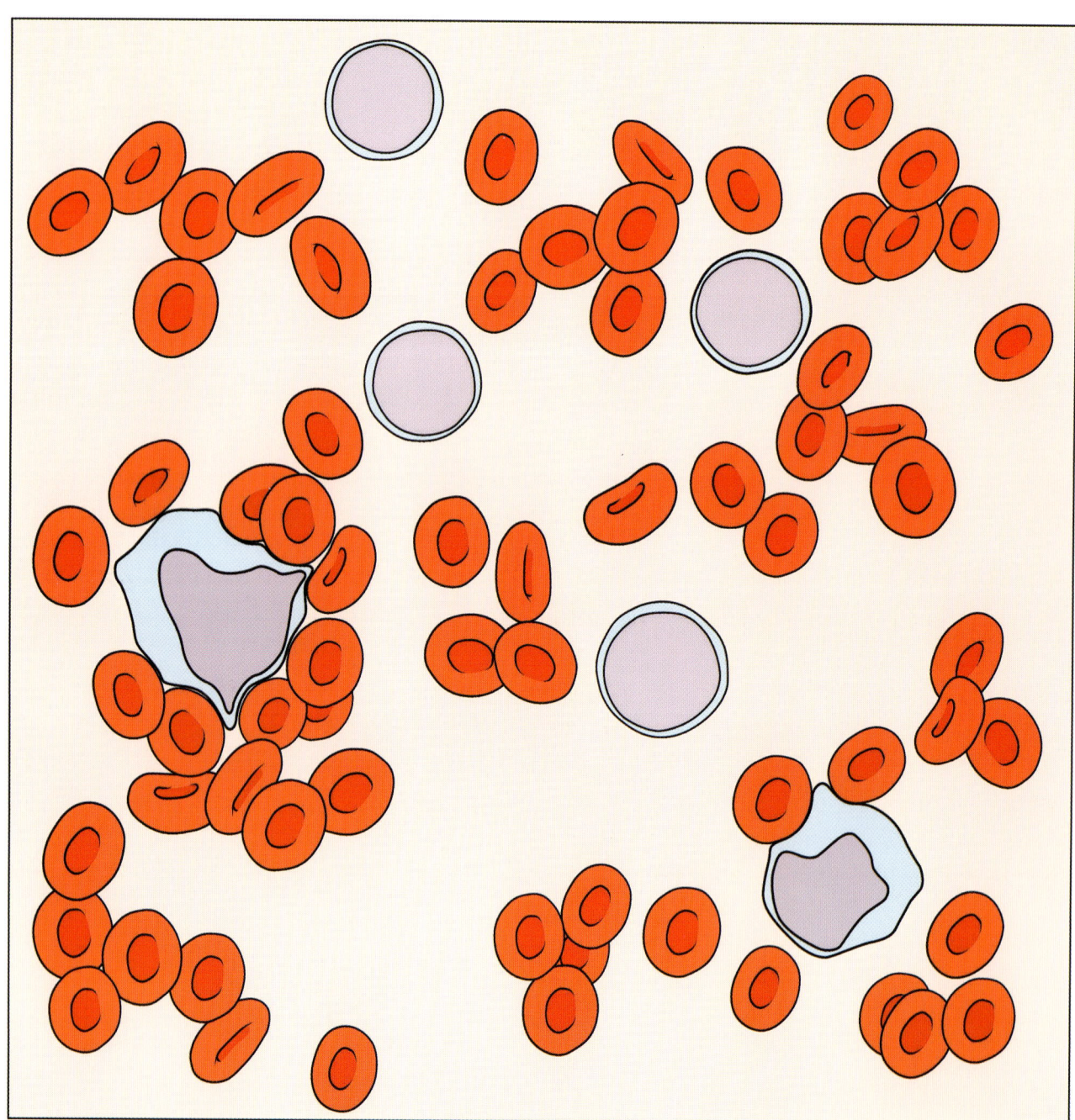

The virus that causes mono affects the lymphocytes in blood (part of the immune system), causing them to be abnormally shaped, as shown in this drawing.

Infectious Mononucleosis

INFECTIOUS MONONUCLEOSIS	
usual age	15 to 25 years
incubation period	30 to 50 days
fever	irregular: usually about 2 weeks
sore throat	marked: whitish-gray exudate
adenopathy (enlargement of lymph nodes)	most commonly anterior and posterior cervical chains; often generalized
splenomegaly (enlargement of spleen)	approximately 50%
hepatomegaly (enlargement of liver)	approximately 10%

words, they are carriers of HHV-4, but they do not have infectious mononucleosis. When illness does develop, however, it is usually exhausting, persistent, and long lasting. Furthermore, since the symptoms can so closely mimic those of the common cold or flu, many people with the condition will go weeks or longer before seeing a doctor or receiving an accurate diagnosis. A definitive diagnosis can only be made through a blood test.

The virus that causes mononucleosis is usually spread through **saliva**, making kissing, sharing food, and sharing utensils all common means of transmission. Its transmission is difficult to control because the first symptoms of illness usually do not appear for a month or more after initial infection. All this time, the infected individual may feel fine, but may still be passing the virus on to others. The virus is commonly spread among children, but children don't usually develop severe illness and are therefore rarely diagnosed with the disease. The actual development of mononucleosis is much more common in teenagers and young adults.

Once a person develops infectious mononucleosis, he can expect to have the symptoms for 1 to 2 months. For the first 1 to 2 weeks, there will be flu-like symptoms including **fever**, body aches, **sore throat**, and swollen lymph nodes. The disease's initial symptoms usually pass after the first week or two, but fatigue is likely to wear on for another 4 to 8 weeks. Usually the body eventually fights off the illness, although the virus will forever exist inside the body, with a small risk of the illness recurring again in the future. Some people with compromised **immune systems**, however, will be much more severely affected and have greater difficulty recovering. Occasionally, mononucleosis can also have fatal complications. For example, infectious mononucleosis sometimes causes severe swelling of an internal organ called the **spleen**. The spleen may become so swollen that it ruptures. A ruptured spleen is dangerous because it can cause severe infection. In some cases, such an infection could ultimately prove fatal. Severe infection, complications, or fatalities, however, are very rare in infectious mononucleosis. With rest and medication to alleviate uncomfortable symptoms, most people make a full recovery and never suffer a relapse of the disease.

For more information, visit Medline Plus at: www.nlm.nih.gov/medlineplus/ency/article/000591.htm

INFERTILITY

Infertility is the inability to reproduce by natural means. The causes of infertility generally lie in the female's **reproductive system**, the male's reproductive system, or the physiological incompatibility of two individuals. There are different treatment options depending on the underlying cause of infertility.

INFLUENZA

Influenza is a family of highly infectious **viruses** that affect the **respiratory system**. Commonly called "the flu," these viruses affect people all over the world, mutate rapidly, and are responsible for a huge amount of lost productivity (from people being unable to attend work or school due to illness) and a significant number of fatalities worldwide every year. Influenza viruses also infect mammals and birds, and sometimes the viruses can mutate and jump from one species to another. The most common cross-species spread occurs between birds, pigs, and humans, most often on farms where these species live in close proximity.

Influenza commonly causes **sore throat**, **fever**, a **cough**, **headache**, and general muscle and body aches. Most people recover relatively quickly and easily. However, the very young, the elderly, and people with compromised **immune systems** are all at increased risk for dangerous complications and fatality. When serious complications arise, it is usually because the influenza has caused **pneumonia**, inflammation and fluid buildup in the **lungs**. When a person has pneumonia, it becomes difficult to breathe and difficult for the lung tissue to absorb **oxygen** as it should—even if air is getting into the lungs, the oxygen may not actually be getting absorbed into the bloodstream.

Certain strains of influenza are more dangerous than others, and throughout history there have been "killer" strains that have caused pandemics (diseases that are geographically widespread and affect a large percentage of that area's population),

DID YOU KNOW?
The 1918–1919 influenza pandemic killed an estimated 50–100 million people around the world—a much higher loss of life than what occurred during World War I.

with high fatality rates, even in healthy individuals. Pandemics generally arise when a new influenza strain appears. New strains are often the result of cross-species leaps. Sometimes influenza strains cross from other animals into people but do not spread easily from person to person. This, so far, has been the case with a particularly deadly form of influenza called H5N1, a subtype that occurs mainly in birds. If a strain cannot spread easily from person to person, it will not cause a worldwide pandemic. When such a strain mutates, however, allowing it

Influenza

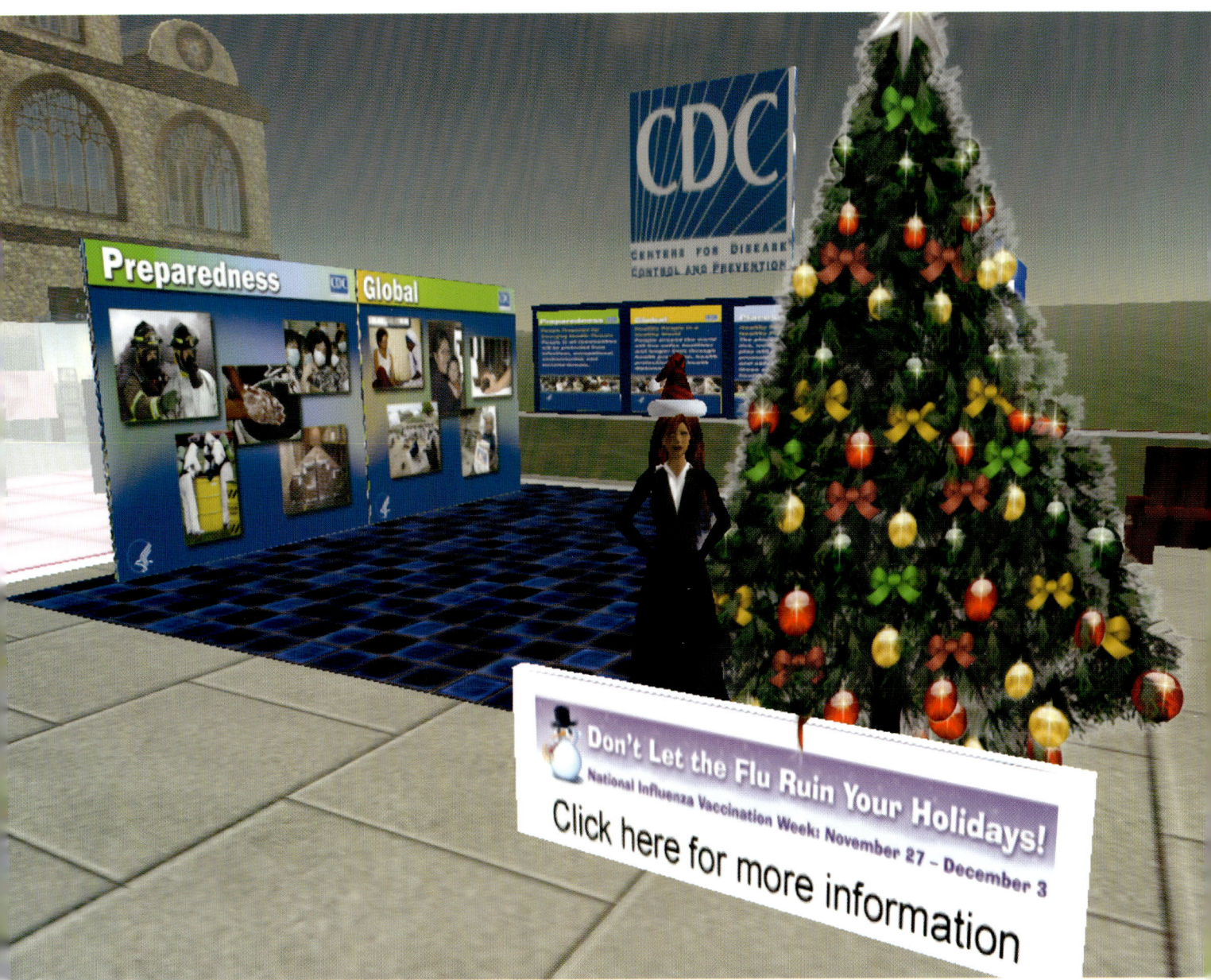

The U.S. Centers for Disease Control and Prevention (CDC) have an informational campaign against the flu. The CDC recommends that people "take 3": Take time to get a vaccine. Take everyday actions to stop germs like frequent hand washing and covering coughs and sneezes. Take antiviral drugs if your doctor says you need them.

to spread easily among people, a pandemic can result. Since humans don't have any resistance to a new influenza strain, it generally proves to be particularly deadly.

The most common means of transmission of influenza viruses is droplet spread. When people cough and *sneeze*, infected *mucus* and *saliva* droplets enter the air. They can then be inhaled by other people, or they can settle on people and surfaces. If they are then transferred into the body, such as by eating food with contaminated hands, that person will also get the infection. Once a person has the flu, she generally must rely on treating the symptoms to maximize comfort until the body fights off the infection. Some

29

Influenza

Weekly Influenza Surveillance Report (12/27/2007-1/5/2008)					
Prepared by the Influenza Division of the CDC					
Data cumulative for the season					
	Influenza Strain				
Region	A (H1)	A (H3)	A Unsub-typed	B	Pediatric Deaths
Nation	307	94	1051	222	1
New England	12	1	36	14	0
Mid-Atlantic	8	2	32	34	0
East North Central	33	20	6	30	0
West North Central	6	3	34	14	0
South Atlantic	19	15	194	46	0
East South Central	2	1	2	0	0
West South Central	17	40	558	29	1
Mountain	130	5	131	39	0
Pacific	80	7	58	16	0

The CDC closely monitors flu cases in the United States. This chart shows how many cases occurred in the various U.S. regions over the course of a single week.

ASK THE DOCTOR

What is an epidemic? How is it different from a pandemic?

A: An epidemic is the emergence of a new infectious disease in a human population at rates much higher than what would normally be expected. A pandemic is an epidemic on a much larger scale—today, "pandemic" usually refers to a global epidemic.

---

antiviral drugs can be used to fight influenza, but to be most effective they must be given as soon as symptoms appear. This generally proves impractical and is only used if a person is at a high risk of developing complications, or if there is a particularly dangerous influenza virus going around. In the next influenza pandemic, antiviral drugs will probably play a large role in treatment, but during the average flu season, they are not widely used.

So far, the best "treatment" for influenza has proven to be prevention. When proper containment and **hygiene** measures are taken, influenza proves to be quite preventable. The first line of defense is frequent and proper hand washing and disinfecting of surfaces that are likely to have been contaminated. It is also important for people with flu symptoms to minimize the risk of passing the illness to others. People with symptoms of influenza should stay home from work or school, take care to always cover their mouth and nose when they sneeze or cough (with a handkerchief or the inside of their elbow, not with the hands, which most readily transfer infected droplets to other locations), and wash their hands frequently and disinfect surfaces that they touch. A combination of responsible behaviors practiced by infected individuals and preventative measures taken by uninfected individuals leads to a huge drop in influenza transmission. Physicians often recommend annual flu shots for individuals who are at greater risk of contracting influenza or who may become more seriously ill if they do contract it.

Flu

"Flu" is a term people commonly use to refer to influenza. People also use the term to refer to other illnesses, such as illnesses of the gastrointestinal tract that cause **nausea**, vomiting, and fever. Sometimes people refer to such an illness as the "stomach flu." This, however, is a misnomer because influenza viruses do not cause gastrointestinal illnesses at all. Occasionally, children with influenza may have nausea or vomiting, but this is caused by other symptoms, such as fever and excess mucus being swallowed and upsetting the stomach. In *gastroenteritis*, in contrast, the nausea and vomiting is caused by infection in the gastrointestinal tract.

INHALANTS

Inhalants are substances inhaled into the respiratory system for the purpose of achieving a "high." Inhalants, including volatile solvents, gases, and nitrites, can be sniffed, huffed, bagged, or snorted. Inhalants are dangerous *drugs*, in part because they can be found in common household products, such as glue, cleaning products, or paint. In fact, this easy accessibility, combined with low cost, and legality makes inhalants one of the first substances abused by children.

Categories of Inhalants include:

- aerosols–sprays containing propellants and solvents, such as spray paints, spray deodorant, and hair sprays
- volatile solvents–liquids that vaporize at room temperature, such as paint thinners, gasoline, glues, and felt-tip markers
- gases–medical anesthetics, such as ether, chloroform, or nitrous oxide; or household products, such as butane lighters, whipped cream bottles, or propane
- nitrites–affect blood vessels, and relax muscles; used as sexual enhancers; commonly known as "poppers" or "snappers"; banned now, but used to be found in video head cleaner or liquid aroma

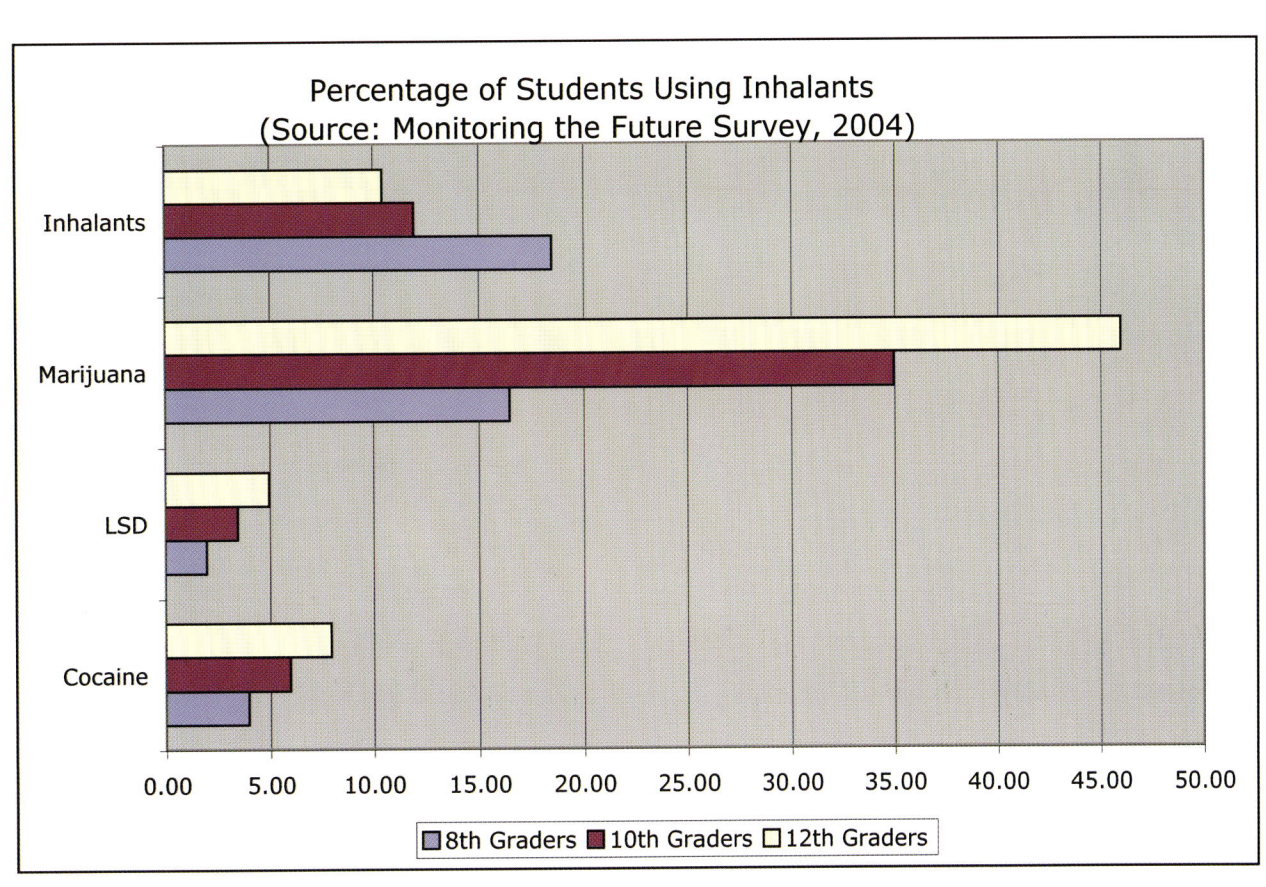

Inhalants

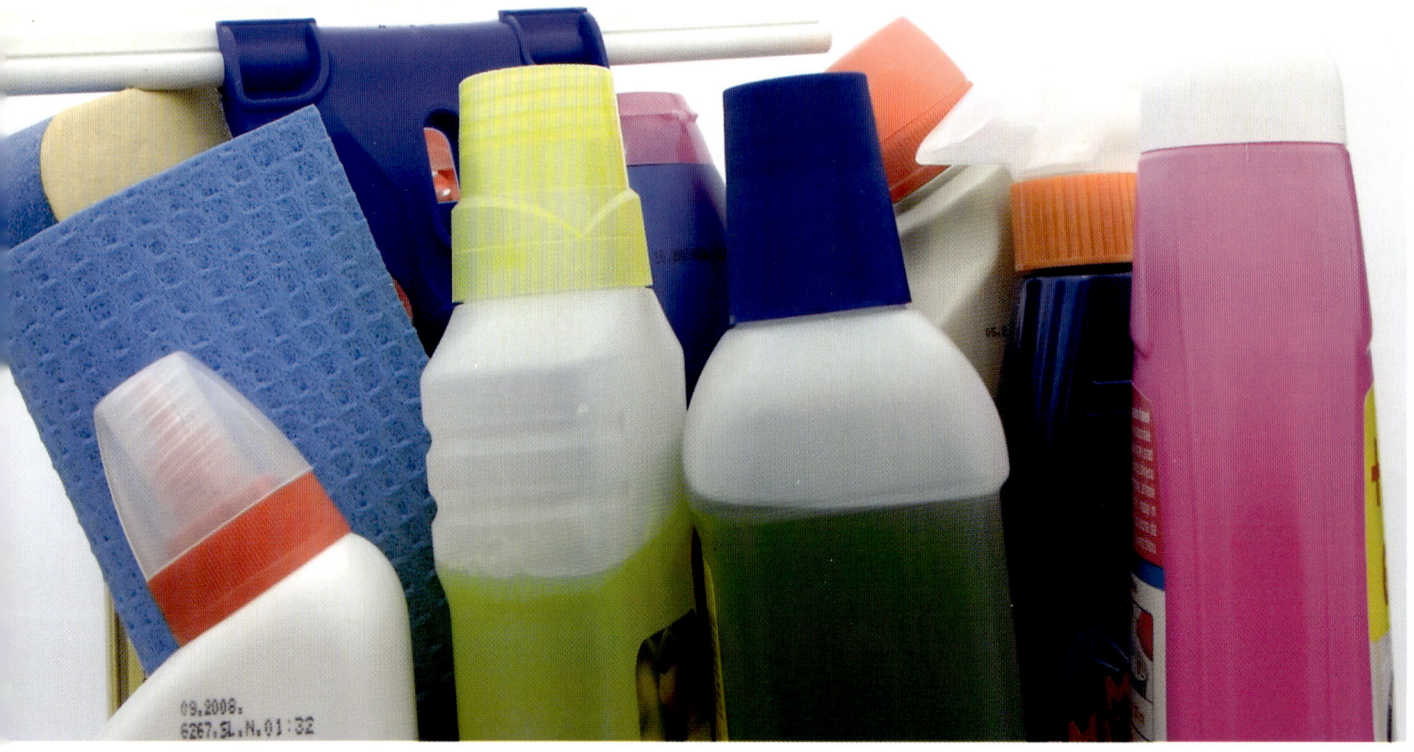

Unlike drugs such as heroin and cocaine, inhalants are easily accessible, since they are the ordinary products found in most households.

Effects of Inhalant Abuse

Inhalants, with the exception of nitrites, act on the central **nervous system** to produce mind-altering (psychoactive) effects. Within seconds after inhalation, the chemicals are absorbed into the bloodstream and travel to the **brain** and other organs. This leads to alcohol-like intoxication, including slurred speech, loss of coordination, dizziness, euphoria, and possibly **hallucinations** or delusions. Prolonged sniffing of the concentrated chemicals can result in rapid, irregular heartbeat and then heart failure and death within just minutes of inhaling. Called "sudden sniffing death," this can occur from a single episode of inhalant use. Chronic use of inhalants can cause memory impairment and **weight** loss, as well as damage to the **heart**, **liver**, **lungs**, and **kidneys**.

Because of the danger of dependence, early intervention is important to stop the abuse before it has serious health consequences. Individuals who are abusing inhalants can be recognized by a number of signs, including chemical odors on breath or on clothing; paint stains on clothing, face, or hands; hidden empty solvent containers or chemical-soaked rags; intoxicated appearance; slurred speech; nausea or appetite loss; and inattentiveness, loss of coordination, irritability, or depression.

Legal Regulation of Inhalants

Inhalants are not regulated under the Controlled Substances Act. However, many states have attempted to prevent youth abuse by placing age restrictions on the sale of certain products. Some states also have made the possession, sale, or distribution of inhalants punishable by fine, incarceration, or mandatory treatment.

For more information, visit the National Inhalant Prevention Coalition at: www.inhalants.org

INSOMNIA

Insomnia is the inability to achieve or maintain sleep. More than one-third of adults in the Western world will experience occasional insomnia, while about one in ten experiences chronic insomnia. It is most common among women and older adults. Each person's experience of insomnia is unique. Some people with insomnia cannot fall asleep quickly when they get into bed. Other people fall asleep easily, but awake in the middle of the night. Still others experience both problems. Whatever the specific problem, the end result is poor-quality sleep that can cause fatigue, moodiness, and difficulty focusing during the day.

Types of Insomnia and Their Causes

Transient insomnia is the inability to sleep well over a period of time lasting fewer than 4 weeks. It is often the result of **stress**, excitement, illness, or physical activity close to bedtime.

Intermittent or short-term insomnia lasts for a period of four weeks to six months, and may come and go. Ongoing stress at work or home, medical conditions, or psychiatric illness can result in the sleep troubles.

Chronic insomnia, or poor sleep most nights for more than 6 months, afflicts more than 20 million people in the United States alone. Chronic insomnia may be primary (not related to another health problem), or secondary (caused by a medical condition).

Diagnosis and Treatment

Determining the cause of insomnia can help diagnose the type and aid in treatment. You and your doctor should discuss both the daytime and nighttime factors that might be disrupting your sleep patterns. Recording your daily routine, your sleep patterns, and how you feel during the day in a sleep diary may also be helpful. In addition to this, your doctor will probably perform a physical exam and take a medical history and a sleep history. In some cases, your doctor may recommend you to a sleep center for further testing.

DID YOU KNOW?

Some people suffering from insomnia actually spend too much time in bed. Instead of lying there hour after hour, trying to fall asleep, they may do better with a sleep restriction program that at first allows only a few hours of sleep a night. Gradually, they can increase their time in bed until they achieve a more normal night's sleep.

Insomnia

Treatment of insomnia will depend on the type. Occasional bouts of insomnia, like those caused by jet lag or stress about a big math test, will resolve once your schedule reverts to normal. Treatment for chronic insomnia will involve reviewing your daily routines for possible causes, and then changing these behaviors when possible. Sleeping pills may also be an option, though side effects and risks should be thoroughly discussed with a doctor. Finally, a method such as relaxation therapy may be attempted to improve sleep.

Some ways to improve the quality of your sleep:

- Create a regular sleep schedule—go to bed at the same time each night and wake up at the same time each morning.
- Do not take naps after 3 pm.
- Avoid caffeine, nicotine or alcohol late in the day.
- Exercise regularly during the day—at least 5-6 hours before bedtime.
- Eat dinner at least 2-3 hours before bedtime.
- Keep your bedroom dark and quiet.
- Write out a to-do list before getting into bed so you won't lay awake worrying about things.
- See your doctor if you think you might have insomnia.

For more information, visit the National Heart Lung and Blood Institute at: www.nhlbi.nih.gov/health/dci/Diseases/inso/inso_whatis.html

INSULIN

Insulin is a hormone made inside the **pancreas**. The pancreas secretes insulin to help

DID YOU KNOW?

During pregnancy, some women develop insulin resistance similar to type 2 diabetes. Known as gestational diabetes, the resulting increase in blood glucose levels can cause birth complications, increased risk of childhood obesity for the child, and development of type 2 diabetes in the woman after pregnancy. The condition can usually be controlled or even reversed with diet modification and exercise.

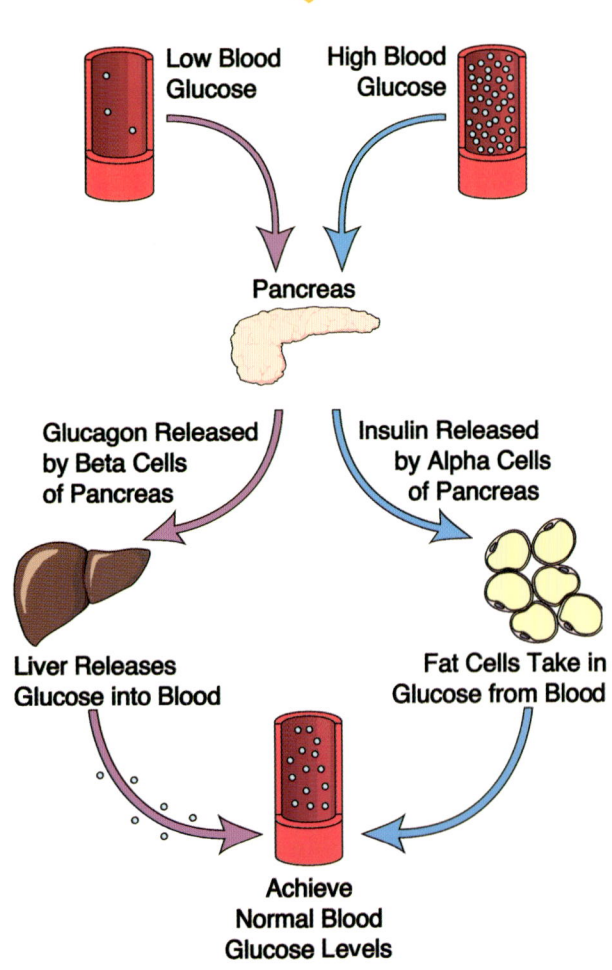

34

Internal Examination

the body use and store the glucose carried into the bloodstream through the ingestion of food. People with type 1 **diabetes** do not create insulin, and must take insulin shots to use the glucose from meals. People with type 2 diabetes do create insulin, but their bodies do not respond correctly to it. In order to obtain energy from the glucose in their meals, they must also receive shots of insulin.

INTERNAL EXAMINATION

An internal examination is an examination of organs and tissues that are inside the body. The term is usually used to refer to a gynecological exam, also called a pelvic exam, in which the **vagina**, **cervix**, **uterus**, **fallopian tubes**, **ovaries**, and **rectum** are examined.

A pelvic exam usually consists of three parts. After an external evaluation is performed, the internal pelvic exam begins with a visual examination and **Pap test**. An instrument called a speculum is used to open the vagina, and a swab is taken of the cervix to test for abnormalities and disease. After this is done, the second part of the pelvic exam takes place. The speculum is removed and the examiner inserts two fingers into the vagina. At the same time, the examiner presses externally on the **abdomen**. In this way, the internal reproductive organs can be evaluated for lumps or other abnormalities. This portion of the pelvic exam is called the "bimanual internal exam." The last part of the pelvic exam is the "rectovaginal exam." While pressing on the abdomen, the examiner inserts one finger into the vagina and one finger into the rectum, again feeling for lumps or other physical abnormalities.

It is highly recommended that all girls and women who have been sexually active for three years or are twenty-one years old or older have yearly internal exams with Pap tests. A yearly internal exam and Pap test is an important part of women's health care,

ASK THE DOCTOR

I'm turning twenty-one soon, and I know this means I should have my first internal exam, but I really don't want to. I feel scared and embarrassed. I don't even want to think about seeing a gynecologist. What should I do?

A: Your feelings are completely normal. Most women experience at least some feelings like yours regarding internal exams. But annual internal exams are an essential part of maintaining good health, so it's important that you find a way to cope with your feelings so you can receive your annual exams. Find a doctor you feel comfortable with. Decide whether you prefer a female or a male doctor. Call some offices, tell them about your feelings, and see if you can meet the doctor before you have the exam. Also, see if any of your friends have had an internal exam yet. If so, ask them what it was like, what their feelings were, and how they dealt with those feelings. Decide whether you'd be more comfortable having someone (like your mother or best friend) with you during the exam, or if you'd be more comfortable alone. Prepare beforehand. Read about internal exams so you know what to expect, and practice relaxation techniques like taking deep breaths and imagining a comfortable place you can mentally retreat to. Finally, remember that the whole exam will be over in a couple of minutes.

Internal Examination

allowing for early detection of diseases, pre-cancerous tissues, and **cancers** of the reproductive system.

For more information visit:
www.youngwomenshealth.org

INTESTINES

The intestines, part of the alimentary canal (the digestive tract), connect the stomach to the anus. They are divided into two major components: the small intestine and the large intestine. Both the small and large intestines share a general structure, and are composed of many layers of tissue. Glands along the interior layer secrete mucus that provides lubrication. The middle and outer layers of tissue are muscle that provides the peristalsis to move food through the intestines.

Small Intestine

The small intestine connects the stomach to the large intestine. The small intestine is coiled up in the abdomen, but if it were straightened out it would stretch for about 21 feet. After the stomach breaks food down into smaller pieces, it sends these pieces into the small intestine. While in the small intestine, the food is broken down even more so that the intestine can extract those nutrients that the body needs to function. Using juices supplied by the pancreas, gallbladder, and liver, the small intestine absorbs the fats, protein, carbohydrates, vitamins, and minerals so that they can enter the bloodstream. Any substances remaining at the end of the small intestine are wastes that are unusable by the body. These wastes are moved along the digestive tract into the large intestine.

Large Intestine

At only about 5 feet, the large intestine, or colon, is shorter than the small intestine. The name comes from the fact that the large intestine is much wider around than the small intestine (3–4 inches vs. 1½–2 inches). The waste products enter the colon still full of liquid. The colon is responsible for extracting and absorbing this water along with any

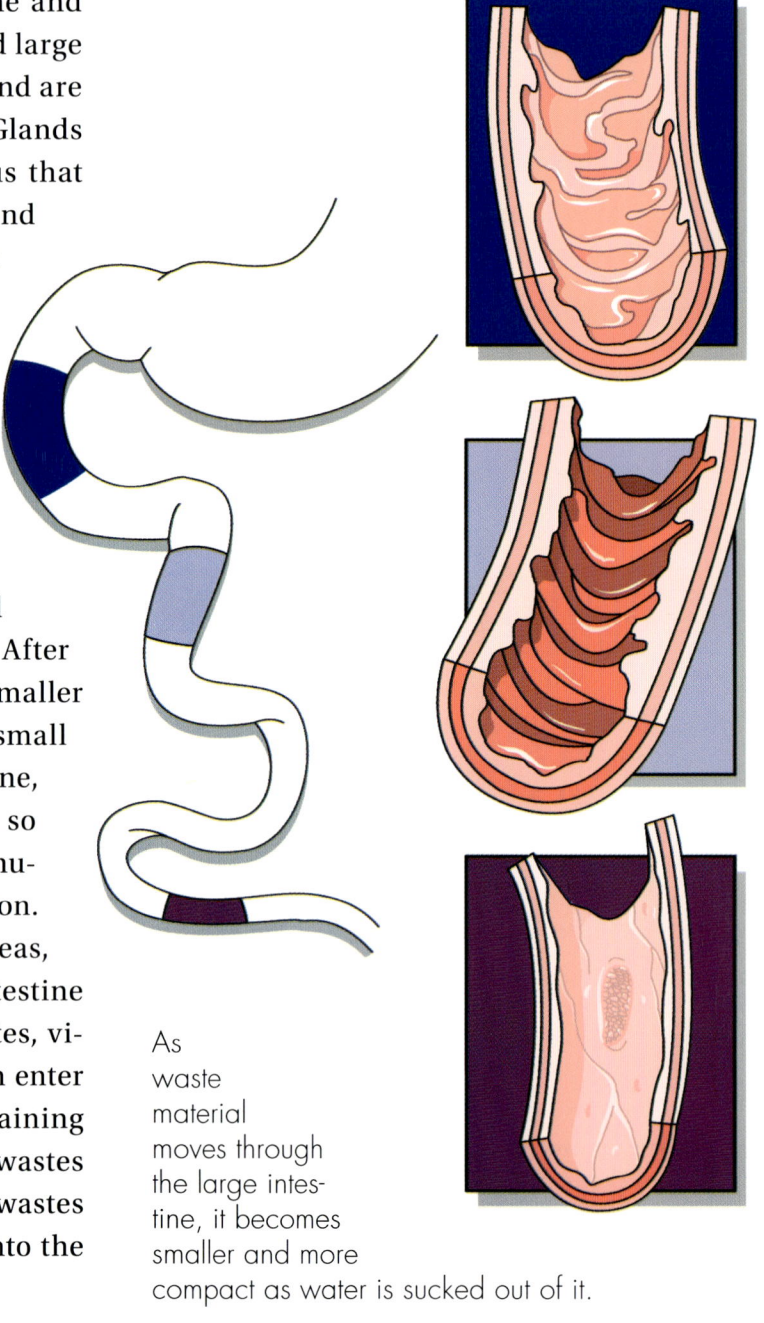

As waste material moves through the large intestine, it becomes smaller and more compact as water is sucked out of it.

36

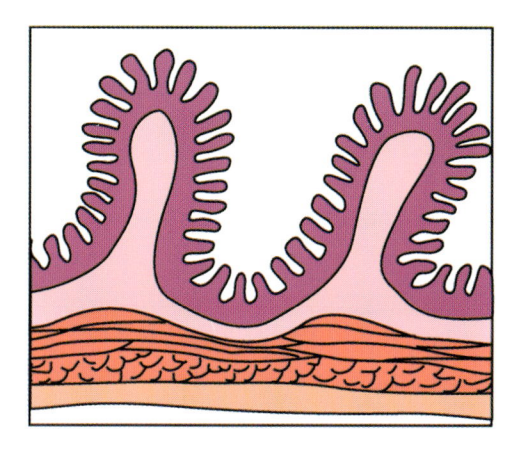

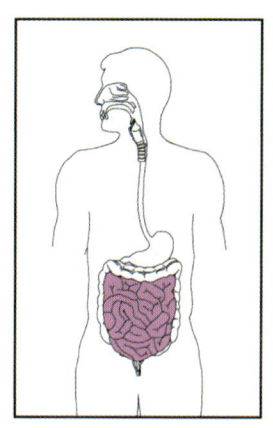

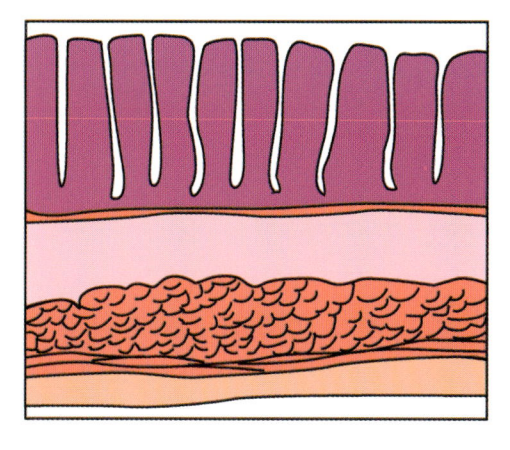

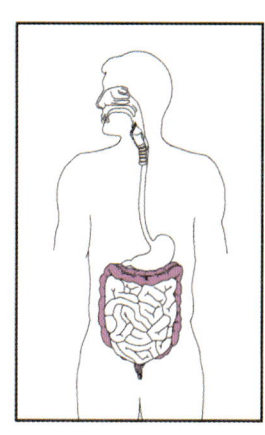

The lining of the small intestine (top) is different from that of the large intestine (bottom). Since the small intestine is the place where most nutrients are absorbed, it needs a huge surface area. The villi, the little finger-like projections shown here, give the small intestine's interior more surface area, and since the material moving through the small intestine is liquid, it is able to flow over and around the villi. Meanwhile, the large intestine's job is primarily to absorb water, and its interior is much smoother so that nothing gets in the way of the solid material moving through it.

remaining minerals. As the waste moves through the large intestine it becomes drier and harder. Eventually, the waste passes from the large intestine into the rectum, where it stays until the body is ready to expel it.

Intestinal Health

The healthy functioning of the intestines is important for overall health, but intestinal problems are one of the most common medical issues. **Diarrhea**, **constipation**, bloating, and abdominal cramps are common intestinal complaints. Most of the time these are passing occur-rences, but chronic problems may be a sign of a more serious problem. Disorders that can affect the intestines include **cancer**, **celiac disease**, **Crohn's disease**, **irritable bowel syndrome**, and bacterial and viral infections, among others. For most people, drinking plenty of water, eating a diet rich in fiber, and leading an active lifestyle will help to maintain healthy intestines.

For more information, visit the National Digestive Diseases Information Clearinghouse at: digestive.niddk.nih.gov/ddiseases/ap.htm

INTOXICATION

Intoxication occurs when a person has consumed, injected, inhaled, or otherwise taken into the body enough of a substance to cause altered or impaired **brain** functioning. This results in a change in mental and/or physical behavior and function. The term intoxication is most commonly used to describe the effects from excessive consumption of alcohol, but it can

DID YOU KNOW?

A 12-oz. bottle of beer, a 5-oz. glass of wine and a 1.5-oz. shot of hard liquor contain the same amount of alcohol.

Intoxication

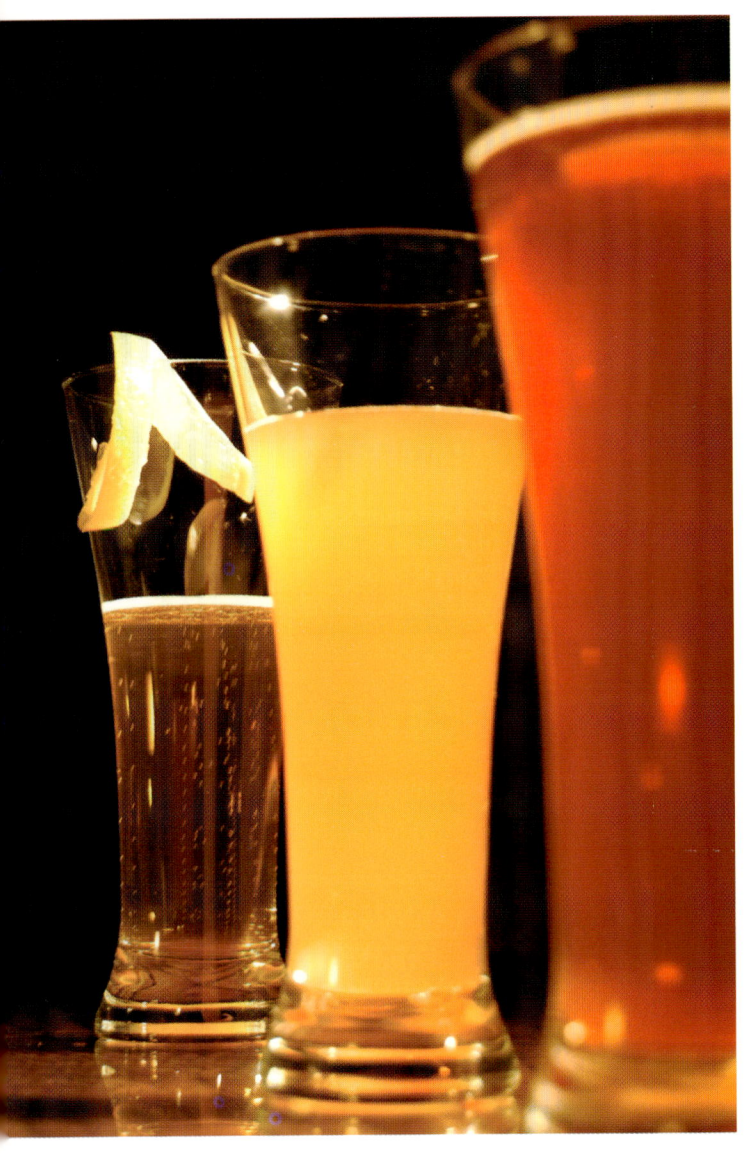

Alcohol abuse and alcohol dependence are not only adult problems; they also affect a significant number of adolescents. According to the U.S. National Institute on Alcohol Abuse and Alcoholism, the average age when boys first try alcohol is 11, while girls' average age is 13. Kids who begin drinking before they are 15 are 4 times as likely to become addicted to alcohol.

be used to describe impairment from any substance. When used in reference to the effects of alcohol, an intoxicated person is often said to be "drunk."

The symptoms an intoxicated individual displays will depend on the substance causing the intoxication. If alcohol is the source, the intoxicated individual will likely display characteristics like exaggerated emotions, slurred speech, and impaired balance and coordination. The individual may also feel more confident than normal, especially in social situations, and experience reduced inhibition. For example, a person who would not normally dance, perform karaoke, or ask someone out on a date might do all those things while intoxicated. The extent to which the individual's behavior and physical abilities are altered will depend on the level of intoxication. Severe intoxication can lead to death.

Binge Drinking

Binge drinking that leads to intoxication is a pattern of excessive alcohol consumption common in the United States, especially on college campuses. The National Institute of Alcohol Abuse and Alcoholism (NIAAA) defines binge drinking as a pattern of drinking that brings a person's *blood* alcohol concentration (BAC) to .08 grams percent or more. Binge drinking has occurred if a man consumes more than 4 drinks or a woman more than 3 drinks in about 2 hours time.

According to the Centers for Disease Control and Prevention (CDC):

- 92% of adults in the United States report binge drinking in the last 30 days.
- 70% of binge drinking involves adults over age 25.
- The rate of binge drinking in men is 3 times the rate in women.
- Binge drinkers are 14 times more likely to drive while under the influence of alcohol.
- Binge drinking accounts for 90% of the alcohol consumed by underage drinkers.

Binge drinking can lead to many unintended consequences and health problems, including injuries, **pregnancy**, **sexually transmitted infections**, alcohol poisoning, brain damage, and death.

IN VITRO FERTILIZATION

Couples that have been unable to conceive naturally use in vitro fertilization (IVF) to have a chance at establishing a **pregnancy**. The woman takes medications designed to stimulate superovulation, or the release of multiple **eggs** at once. The use of multiple eggs increases the chance of eventual success. Once the eggs are retrieved, they are combined with **sperm** outside of the body. The fertilized eggs are then allowed a few days to develop under controlled laboratory conditions before being transferred to the uterus for potential implantation. Since multiple embryos are transferred to the uterus, IVF increases the chance of a **multiple birth** pregnancy.

IRRITABLE BOWEL SYNDROME

Irritable bowel syndrome (IBS) is a condition of the **digestive system** in which a person experiences pain, bloating, excess gas, and irregular bowel movements and functioning. One of the most common causes of IBS is stress. **Diet** may also play a significant role.

Tips to help control the symptoms of IBS

Eat a varied healthy diet.
Avoid foods high in fat.
Increase the amount of fiber in your diet.
Avoid caffeine and alcohol.
Drink plenty of water.
Try eating several small meals a day rather than 3 larger ones.
Learn healthy stress-management skills.
Avoid using laxatives.

ITCHES

Itches are uncomfortable sensations of the **skin** that produce an urge to scratch. The itchy area may appear irritated or inflamed, or it may have no abnormal appearance at all. Likewise, the itch sensation may have a clear cause, such as a skin **rash** or exposure to a skin irritant, or it may have no discernable cause. Itching is not fully understood by science, but it has been determined that the neurological receptors that detect itch only occur in the skin (itching is not felt by

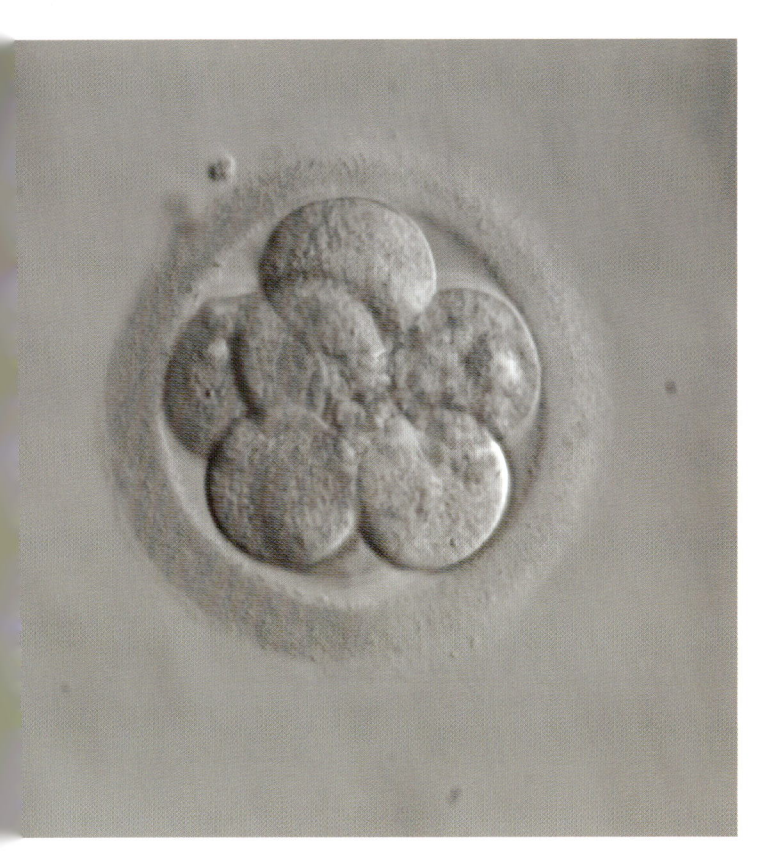

This photo shows a tiny 8-celled embryo ready to be transferred into the uterus.

Itches

other parts of the body like internal organs or **bones**).

Itching appears to have a lot in common with the sensation of **pain**, but is caused by distinct receptors and mechanisms. Quite mysteriously, itching can, like pain, sometimes be felt in limbs or parts of the body that no longer exist. Some amputees or people who have lost limbs or body parts experience a phenomenon called "phantom limb pain" in which they continue to feel pain in the place the body part used to be. They may have this same "phantom" experience with other sensations, including itch.

Itches may be treated in a number of ways. Simple itches are often "cured" by scratching. Scratching, however, can be damaging to the skin, especially for a prolonged or chronic itch, and may be ineffective. Often treating the underlying cause of the itch is the most effective course of action. If, for example, the itch is caused by a fungal infection, treating the fungal infection is the best course of action for permanent itch relief. However, treating the underlying cause of an itch may take a significant amount of time before it relieves the itch—and when you're itchy, you probably don't want to wait that long! In the meantime, itch-inhibiting ointments or medications may be used. Although most itches have a physical cause, some have psychiatric causes. Certain psychiatric disorders, for example, can lead to "tactile hallucinations"—hallucinations in which an individual perceives a physical sensation (like itching) that is not physically present (the itch receptors are not stimulated). In these situations, physical remedies will not cure the itch because the itch does not have a physical cause.

Jaundice

JAUNDICE

Jaundice is a yellowing of the **skin**, the whites of the **eyes**, or **mucus** membranes. The yellow color is caused by bilirubin, which is a byproduct of dying red **blood** cells. Each day, about 1% of our red blood cells retire to be replaced by new ones. The old red blood cells are processed by the **liver** and leave the body as waste. Much of the bilirubin created in this process also leaves the body with other solid waste. However, if too many red blood cells retire at once, or the liver is malfunctioning, the bilirubin builds up in the body. Eventually, the build-up results in jaundice.

Infant Jaundice

Many infants have jaundice in the first week after **birth**. Birth is a stressful ordeal for the infant's body, and it causes many red blood cells to retire. The newborn's liver cannot handle the influx of red blood cells, and bilirubin builds up. The infant should be evaluated, but most cases clear up within a week or two following birth. If the jaundice doesn't clear up on its own, the doctor may prescribe ultraviolet light therapy, during which the infant is placed under a special UV light for several days. Other treatments might be necessary is the jaundice is severe, or if it seems to be caused by a more serious underlying condition.

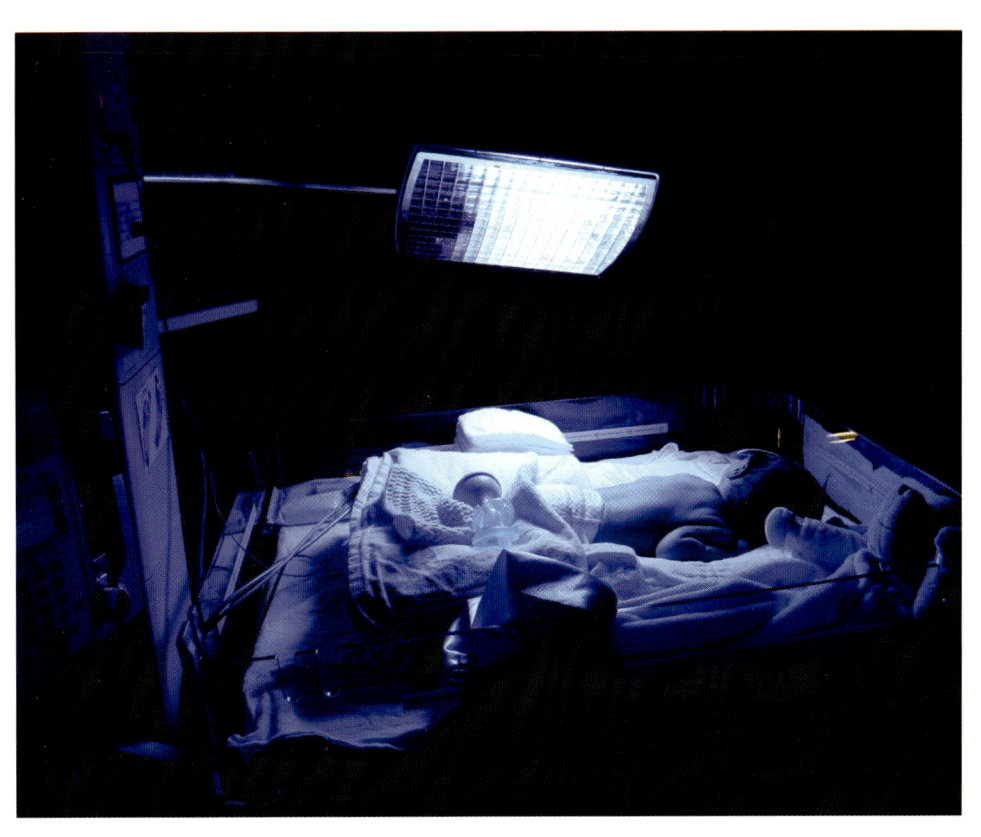

During phototherapy (light treatment), the baby's skin and blood absorb light waves, which break down the bilirubin into substances that can more easily pass through the baby's system.

For more information, visit the Mayo Clinic at: www.mayoclinic.com/health/infant-jaundice/DS00107/DSECTION=1

Joints

JOINTS

Joints are the places in the body where **bones** come together. Many joints have a structure that permits movement, but not all of the body's joints are movable. There are a number of different types of joints in the body, and they are usually classified by their structure and by their function.

> There are three major structural classifications of joints:
> - fibrous/immovable
> - cartilaginous
> - synovial
>
> There are also three major functional classifications of joints:
> - synarthrosis
> - amphiathrosis
> - diarthrosis
>
> Each joint classification can also be divided into further subcategories.

Fibrous/Immovable Joints

These are places where bones are joined in static connections—connections that do not allow movement, where two different bones are essentially fused together with connecting tissues. The skull, for example, has a number of fibrous/immovable joints called sutures. The skull does not move and behaves as if it was one bone, but it is actually made up of different bones joined together.

Cartilaginous Joints

Cartilaginous joints are where a type of tissue called cartilage connects two bones. These joints allow some limited movement, with the cartilage acting as a cushioning pad between the bones. The spine, for example, contains numerous cartilaginous joints. The vertebrae are connected to one another with pads of cartilage called intervertebral discs. Movement of the spine is limited to certain directions, and the amount of movement occurring between each individual vertebra is quite small.

ASK THE DOCTOR

My friend says he's double jointed. What does that mean? Does he actually have two joints where he should only have one?

A: No. The term "double jointed" is used to describe someone with an unusual amount of flexibility in one or more joints. This is caused by very elastic, or stretchy, ligaments. Ligaments are usually quite taut, holding the joints firmly together. "Double-jointed" people have enough flexibility in their joints to make their joints appear to move in unusual ways.

What is that noise when I "crack" my knuckles? Is it bad to do this?

A: A fluid-filled capsule surrounds the moveable joints of your body. The synovial fluid inside the capsule contains nutrients and gases. That sound you hear when you crack your knuckles is the sound of gas bubbles popping as the joint capsule is stretched. Whether or not it is unhealthy is still up for some debate. While there is no evidence that knuckle cracking causes arthritis, some studies do suggest it may damage soft tissue around the joints, cause swelling, and weaken your grip.

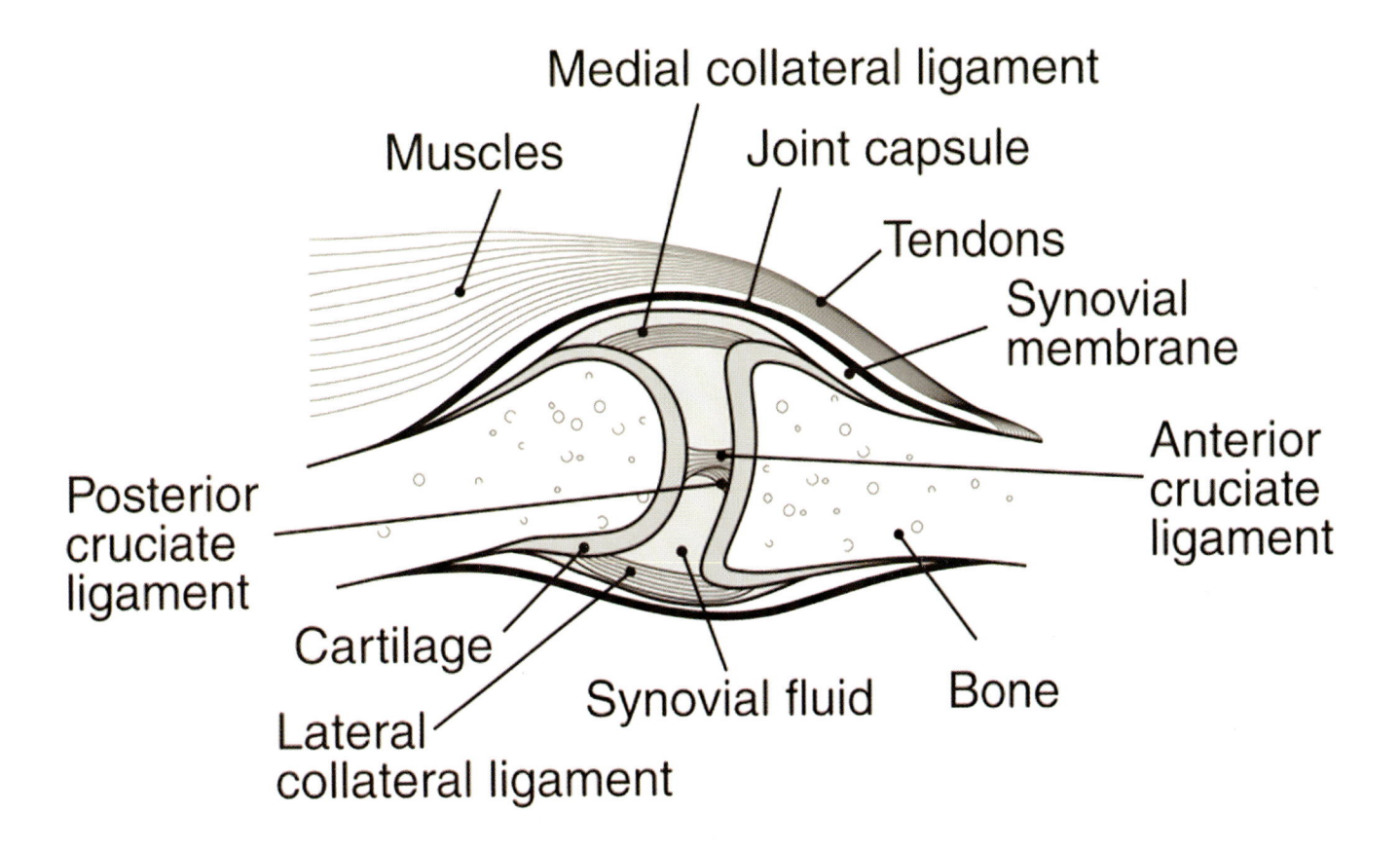

Synovial Joints

Synovial joints are the most mobile joints of the body. They occur where two bones come together in a fluid-filled space. This synovial fluid supports, cushions, and permits a wide range of motion. There are different types of synovial joints. The **hip**, for example, is a type of synovial joint called a ball-and-socket joint because one bone has a round, ball-like end that fits into the other bone's concave, bowl-like socket.

Joint Function and Injury

In addition to structure, joints can also be classified by function—in this case, the type and amount of movement they permit. Joints may display synarthrosis (joining that permits no movement), amphiathrosis (joining that permits some very limited movement), and diarthrosis (joining that permits movement). Synovial joints are the only joints in the body that display diarthrosis.

Mobility is the main purpose of many of the body's joints, but joints serve an additional function by cushioning the bones and absorbing shock. For this reason, they are relatively susceptible to injury. High-impact sports and **exercise** can sometimes damage joints, especially after years of rigorous training and competition. Joint injuries are very common among both professional and nonprofessional athletes. Excess **weight** is also extremely taxing on joints. Even relatively low levels of excess weight can, over the long term, adversely affect the joints. **Obesity** is a very common cause of joint pain and impairment. In most people, the **knee** joints are highly susceptible to injury because they consistently support the full weight of the body on a relatively complex and delicate structure. Excess weight

Joints

and obesity are very common causes of knee pain and injury, as are high-impact sports.

Dislocation

Dislocation occurs when a bone moves out of its normal location in the joint, usually causing *pain* and restricted movement. Dislocation results in stretching and damage to the ligaments that hold the joint in place. Other soft tissues in the joint may also be damaged. Once a joint has become dislocated, it is often more likely to become dislocated again because of stretching of the ligaments. Dislocation usually occurs as the result of a fast, hard impact, such as a vehicular accident or a collision and fall in a sport. It is sometimes possible, however, to suffer a dislocation

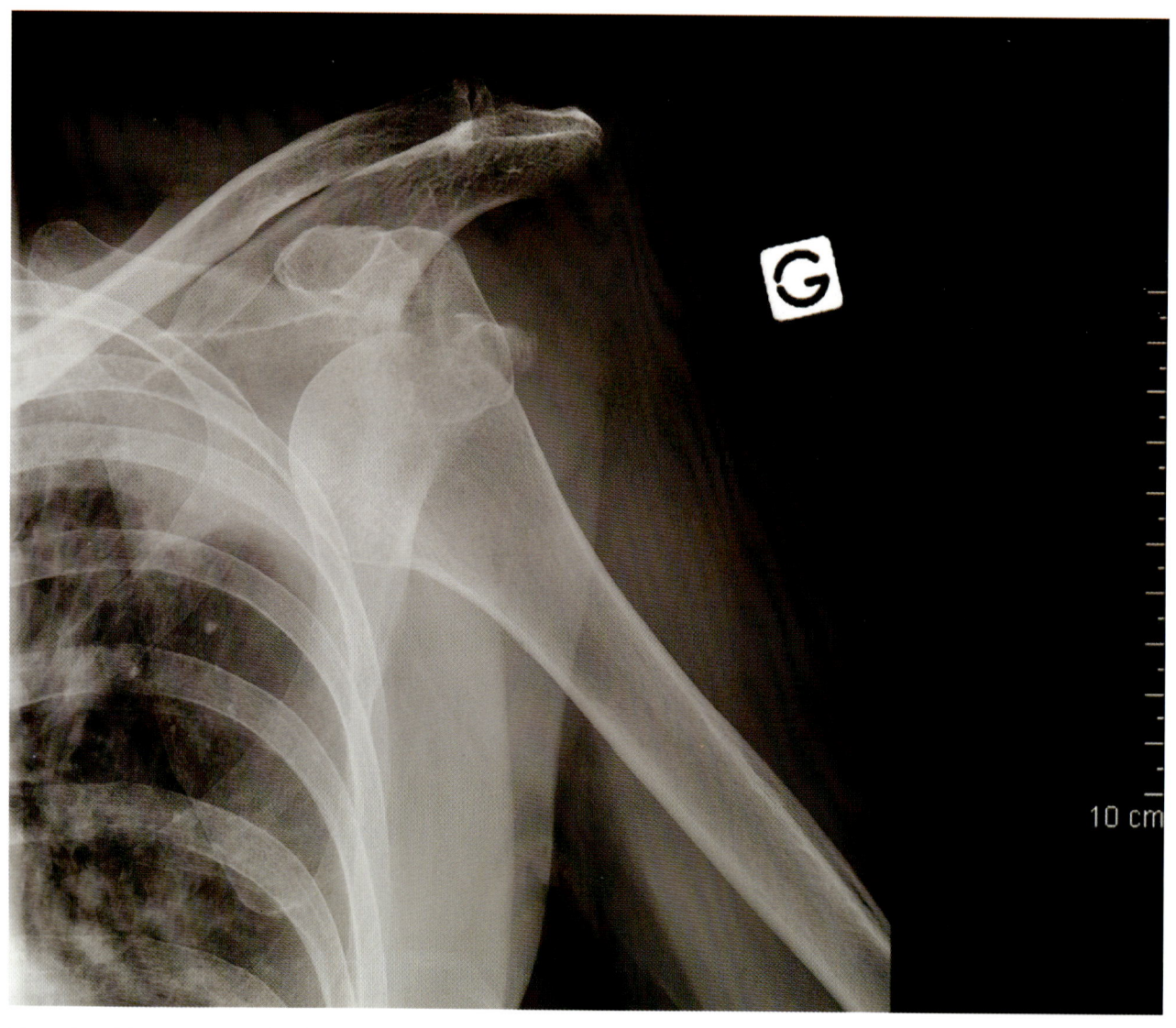

Your shoulders are your body's most mobile joints, but their ability to move in many directions means they are also prone to injury—such as when your upper arm bone pops out of the cup-shaped socket that's part of your shoulder blade (as shown here in this X-ray). A dislocated shoulder requires prompt medical attention, but most people regain full shoulder function within a few weeks. Once you've had a dislocated shoulder, however, your joint may become more prone to dislocation.

Joints

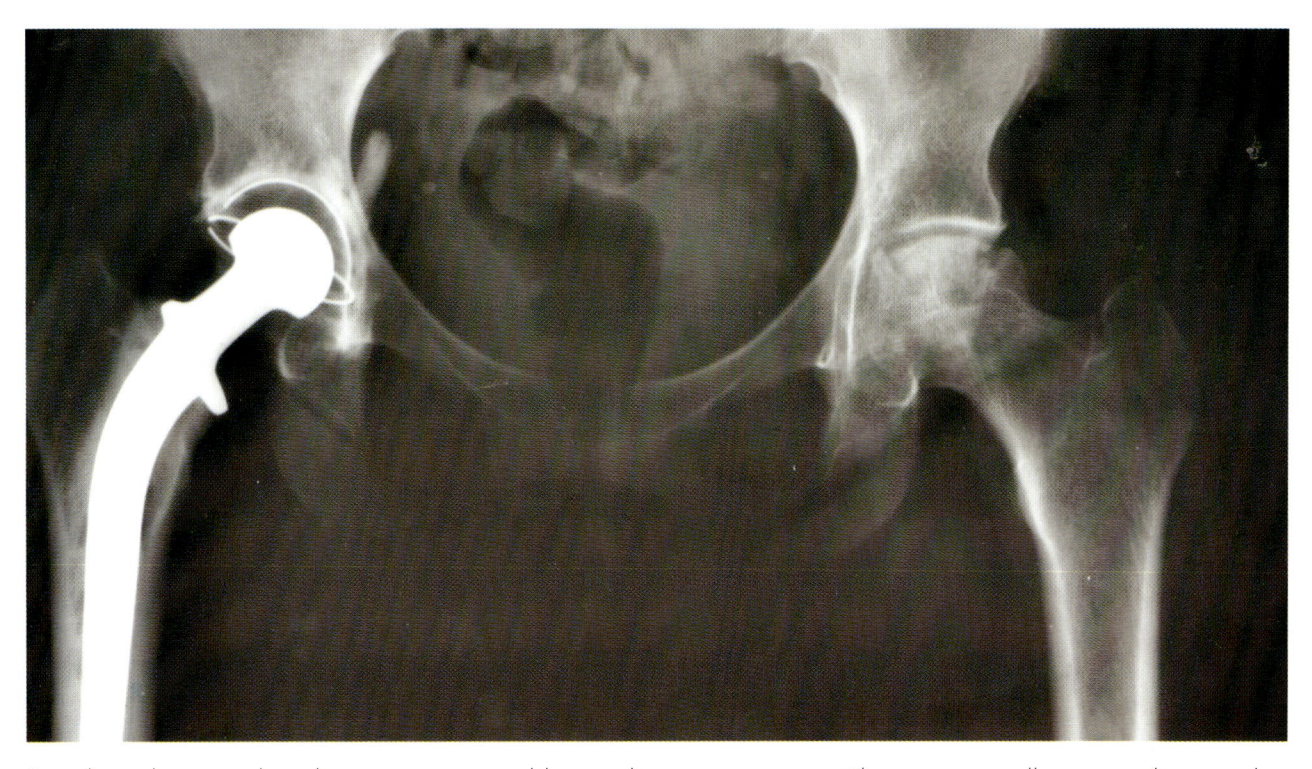

People with severe hip damage may need hip replacement surgery. The surgeon will remove damaged cartilage and bone from the hip joint and replace them with new, man-made parts (as shown here in this X-ray).

through more regular daily activities, but this is usually only the case if the person's joints or ligaments have been severely weakened by disease or previous injuries.

Sometimes dislocated joints promptly return to their normal position on their own. If this does not happen, however, it is important to see a health-care professional who can return the bones to their normal alignment while minimizing additional damage. It may be possible for people to manipulate a dislocated joint back into position without medical aid, but doing so runs a significant risk of causing additional damage to the joint. Once the joint is properly aligned, it may need to be immobilized or stabilized with a splint, brace, or other structure during the healing process. It may also require *physical therapy* to regain strength and reduce the chances of a repeat injury. In some cases, surgery may also be required to repair damaged tissues or prevent repeat injury.

Joint Replacement

Joint replacement is a major surgery to replace part or all of a joint's surfaces with synthetic materials. Joint replacement surgery is extremely common for the knee and hip joints, especially in athletes later in life, people with obesity, and the elderly. Severe *arthritis*, causing degradation of the cartilage that cushions the joint, is the most common cause of severe joint pain and reduced mobility requiring joint replacement surgery. After surgery, physical therapy is required to achieve the best outcome. Overall, joint replacement surgery has very positive results, usually resulting in a great improvement in pain and quality of life. Full mobility, however, cannot always be restored.

Kidneys

K

KIDNEYS

The kidneys are the organs responsible for filtering impurities from the *blood*. These are then flushed from the body as *urine*. The two bean-shaped kidneys are located near the middle of the *back*, just below the rib cage.

Function

The kidneys are responsible for removing waste products from the blood. Blood is carried to the kidneys by the renal artery. Once in the kidneys, the blood moves through tiny filters, called nephrons. The nephrons remove the impurities, combine them with

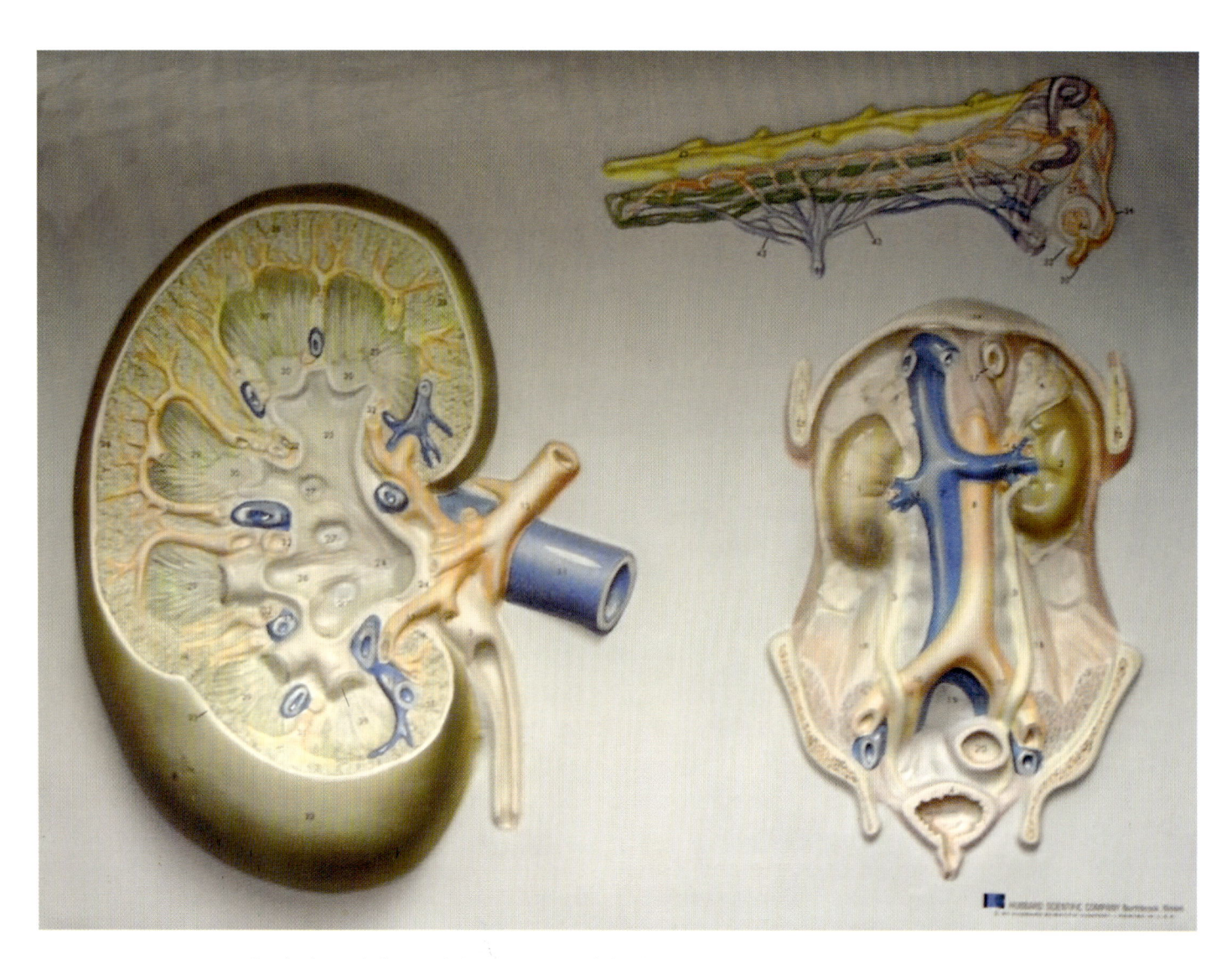

A cross-section of a kidney (left), and the position of the kidneys within the body (right).

Kidneys

> **DID YOU KNOW?**
>
> Each kidney is around 5 inches long or only about the size of a fist, yet your kidneys filter all the blood in your body about 400 times a day!

water to make urine and send them down the ureter and into the **bladder**. The filtered blood is returned into the body through the renal vein.

The kidneys are also responsible for balancing the volume of fluids and minerals in the body. If you are dehydrated, the kidneys will hold on to more water until you take a drink and replenish your fluids. Once you are re-hydrated, the kidneys release the extra fluid as urine. The kidneys also help regulate the level of minerals, such as sodium, phosphorus, and potassium, in the blood stream.

In addition to these functions, the kidneys secrete three important hormones into the body:

- Erythropoietin stimulates bone marrow to make red blood cells.
- Renin regulates blood pressure.
- Cacitriol (active vitamin D) helps maintain calcium for strong bones.

Disorders

When kidneys are not functioning correctly, dangerous levels of waste and fluid can build up in the body. Loss of kidney function is usually the result of a disease that attacks the nephrons and diminishes their filtering ability. Damage can be sudden, perhaps as the result of an injury, but usually the damage happens slowly, over a long period of time. **Diabetes** and high blood pressure are two common causes of kidney disease. Symptoms of kidney disease include frequent urination, loss of appetite, nausea, vomiting, and fatigue. Swollen or numb extremities, drowsiness, and muscle cramps are also signs of kidney malfunction.

Treatment

Chronic kidney disease cannot be cured. However, if you have kidney disease you can extend the life of your kidneys by keeping glucose levels under control, controlling blood pressure levels, and avoiding pain medications. In addition, your doctor may order certain dietary restrictions, such as limiting protein and fat ingestion, and reducing sodium and potassium intake. If kidneys fail completely, the only options are dialysis or kidney transplant. Dialysis is an artificial means of filtering out waste products; there

If you have two healthy kidneys, you have more than you really need. Some people are born with only one kidney, and many people donate a kidney for transplantation to a family member or friend; all these people can lead normal, healthy lives. If you have less than 25 percent of normal kidney function, however, you will have serious health problems.

Kidneys

are two forms. Hemodialysis filters the blood 3 times a week. Each dialysis treatment takes about 3 to 4 hours. During peritoneal dialysis a fluid is put into the abdomen to capture waste products. Every few hours this fluid must be drained and replaced. A kidney transplant involves replacing the failed kidney with one from a donor. The donor may either be a recently deceased individual or a living "match," usually a relative.

For more information, visit the National Institute of Diabetes and Digestive and Kidney Diseases at: kidney.niddk.nih.gov/kudiseases/pubs/yourkidneys/#1

KNEE

The knee is the *joint* that connects the **bone** of the upper leg (the femur) to the bone of the lower leg (the tibia). The knee is a complex structure that is actually made of two joints. It aids in walking, running, and other forms of locomotion. Many types of movement cause most of the body's weight to fall on the knees, making knee injuries very common, especially in high-impact sports. The knee is also one of the joints most commonly affected by **arthritis**.

The two joints that make up the knee are the femoro-patellar joint and the femoro-tibial joint. Both are synovial joints, meaning the bones come together in a fluid-filled space that allows for significant movement. The femoro-patellar joint is where the kneecap meets the femur. The femur has a concave section called the patellar groove that the rounded kneecap nestles and slides along. The femoro-tibial joint is where the femur and the tibia meet.

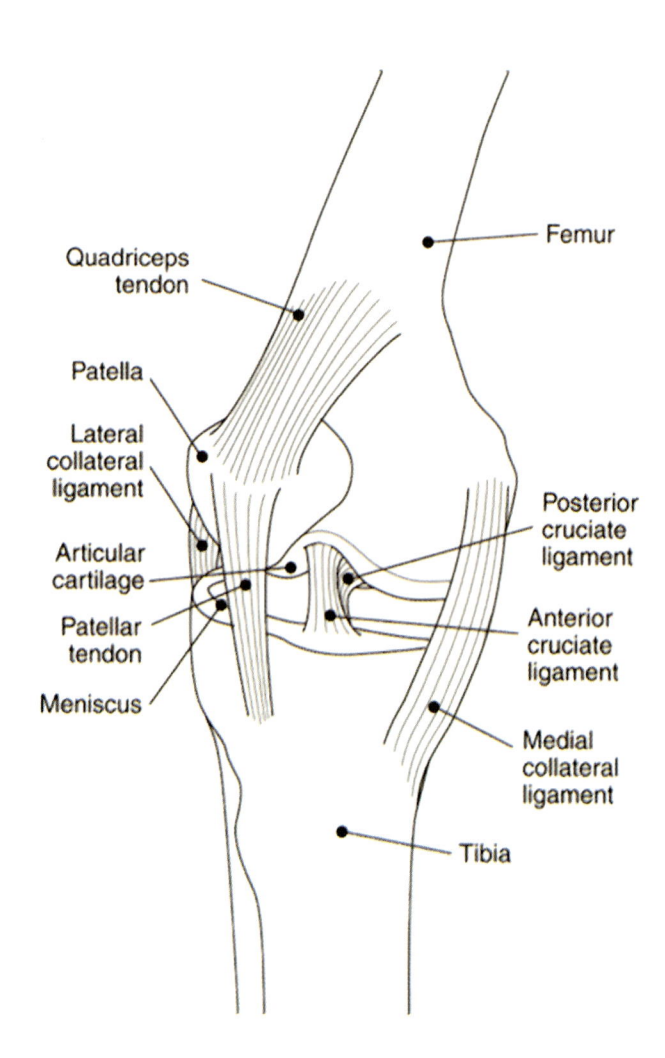

L

LACERATIONS

Lacerations are a type of **skin** wound. There are many ways in which the skin can be injured or opened. People often refer to **cuts** in the skin as "lacerations," but medically speaking, this is incorrect. Whereas cuts usually have "clean" or smooth edges (generally created by a very sharp object like a knife or glass), lacerations are irregular. They are usually caused by tearing of the skin or by blunt-force trauma. Lacerations are often seen on parts of the body where the soft tissue is thinly stretched over hard tissue; the skull and shin are two examples of such locations. Blunt-force trauma to these areas can cause the thin tissue to tear. Lacerations can be minor or severe. Severe lacerations may require **stitches** to hold the tissues together to staunch bleeding and promote healing.

LACTATION

Lactation is the production of milk by the mammary **glands**. This is done for the purpose of feeding an infant, as in **breastfeeding**.

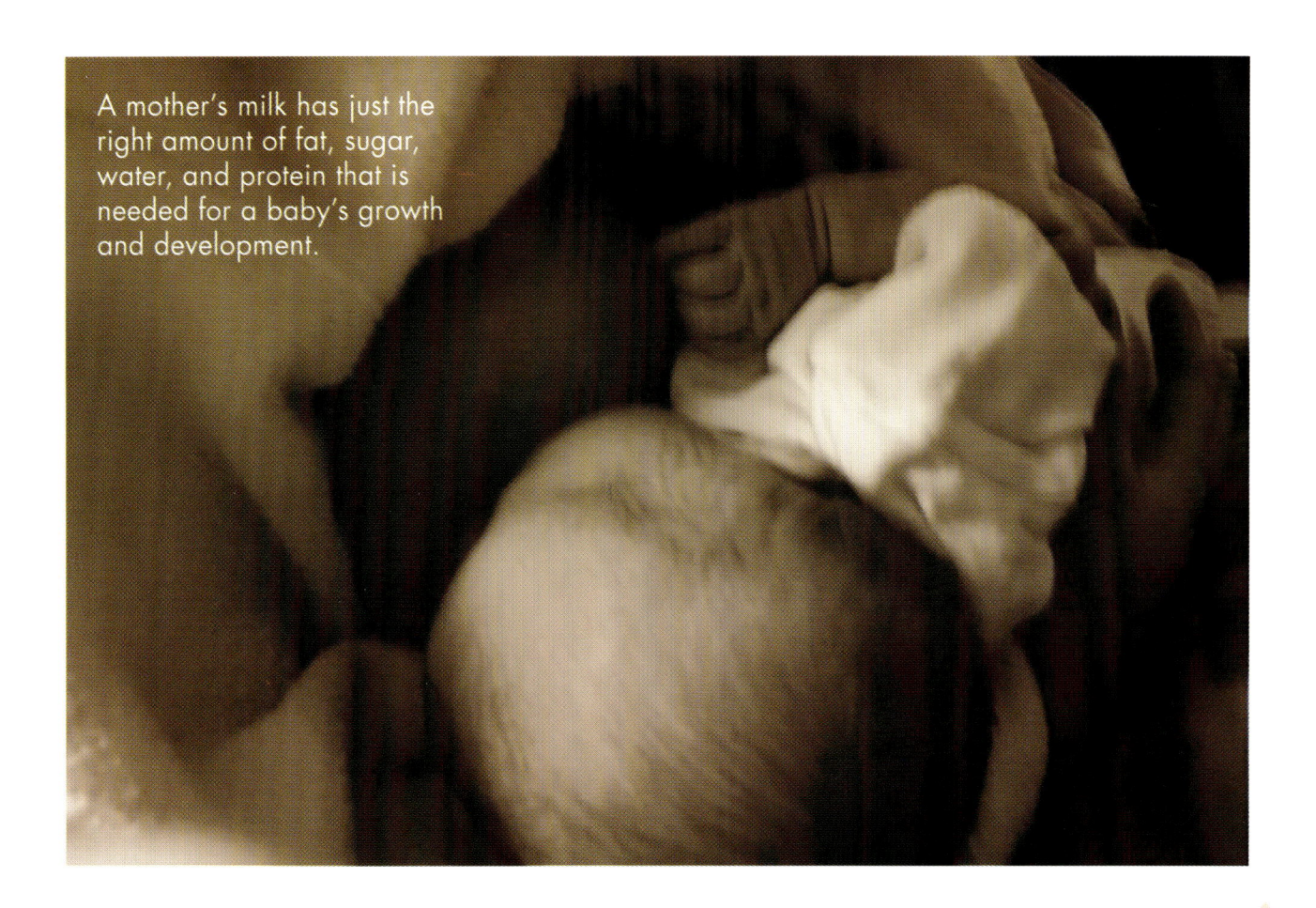

A mother's milk has just the right amount of fat, sugar, water, and protein that is needed for a baby's growth and development.

Larynx & Laryngitis

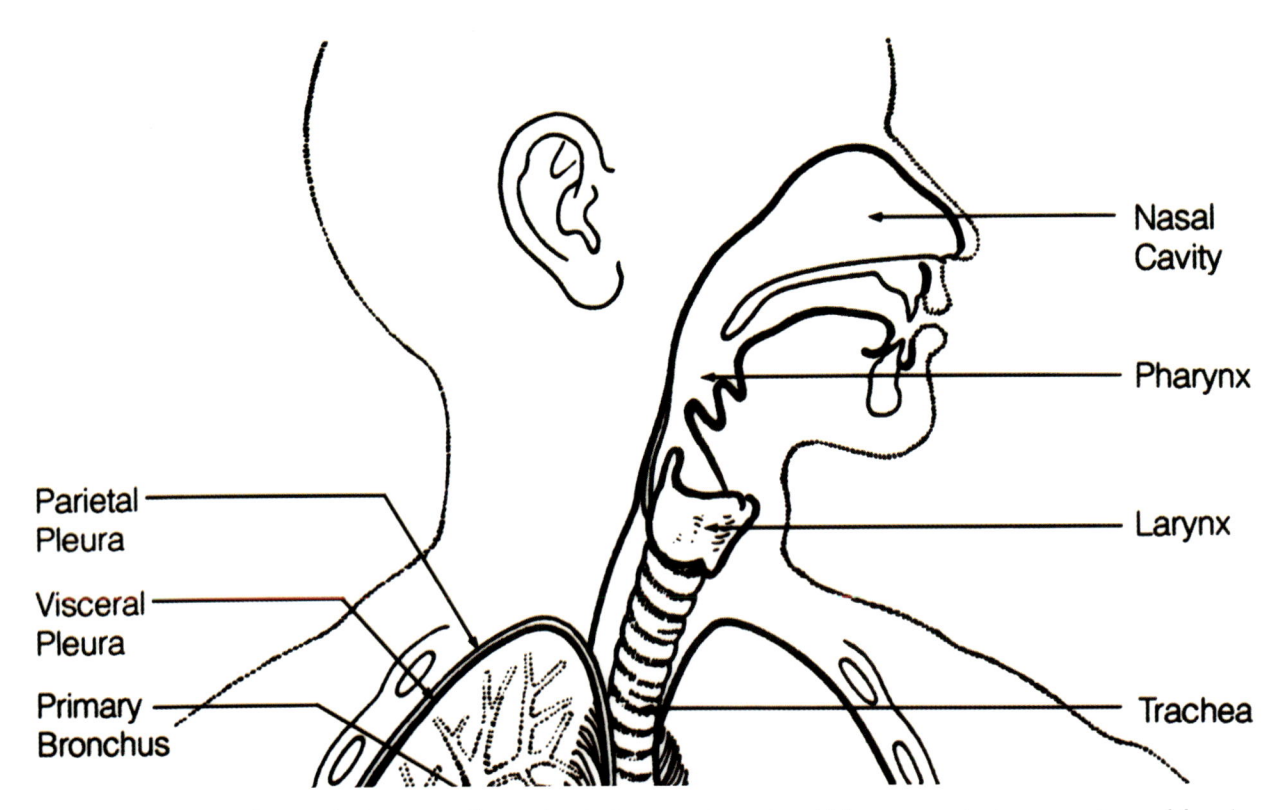

Not only does your larynx help you talk, it also helps you breathe. When you choke on a bite of food, your larynx stimulates a cough reflex, protecting your lungs.

LARYNX AND LARYNGITIS

The larynx, also commonly called the "voice box," is a structure in the **neck** responsible for the production of sound. It also plays a protective role in shielding the trachea (also called the "windpipe"). Sound is produced in the larynx when air is forced from the lungs over the larynx's vocal folds.

Laryngitis

Laryngitis occurs when the larynx becomes irritated and inflamed. This may happen because of improper or overuse of the larynx (a relatively common situation in singers), because of a physical irritant such as **stomach** acid, or because of **infection**. Laryngitis caused by infection can be bacterial or viral. Symptoms of laryngitis include a dry, persistent **cough**, a weak voice or an inability to speak, and a persistent tickling sensation in the throat. The symptoms are made worse by talking and often get more severe at night. Laryngitis is often accompanied by a **sore throat**.

If the laryngitis lasts only a few days, it is called acute. It is quite common, however, for laryngitis to be persistent and drag on for an extended period of time. If it continues for more than 3 weeks, it is called chronic. When laryngitis is chronic, a medical evaluation should be sought to rule out other illnesses and conditions, such as vocal cord nodules and laryngeal **cancer**.

Treatment of laryngitis depends on the cause of the inflammation. If the cause is overuse of the **vocal cords**, rest and steps to relieve discomfort, such as taking a **painkiller** and drinking hot tea, may be all that is required. If the laryngitis recurs, however, it may be a sign that there is a larger problem. If the cause of the laryngitis is bacterial, the body may fight off the infection on its own. If not, an **antibiotic** may be prescribed. If the cause is viral, basically all one can do is rest and treat the symptoms until the body fights off the virus. Finally, if a physical irritant causes the laryngitis, the irritant must be removed for the laryngitis to resolve. The most common irritant to cause laryngitis is stomach acid. Some people with severe acid reflux (also called **heartburn**), may actually have stomach acid flowing up into their throat and damaging the soft tissues of the larynx. This situation can cause permanent damage to the larynx and voice.

LASERS

Lasers are concentrated beams of light. Their name comes from the phrase "light amplification by stimulated emission of radiation." Some lasers are so concentrated and powerful they can be used to burn and cut objects. Lasers are so precise they can be particularly useful in medical applications. Today, lasers are used to perform many types of surgeries and medical procedures. In addition to being precise, they cause extreme heat at the site of cutting. This also has a very useful

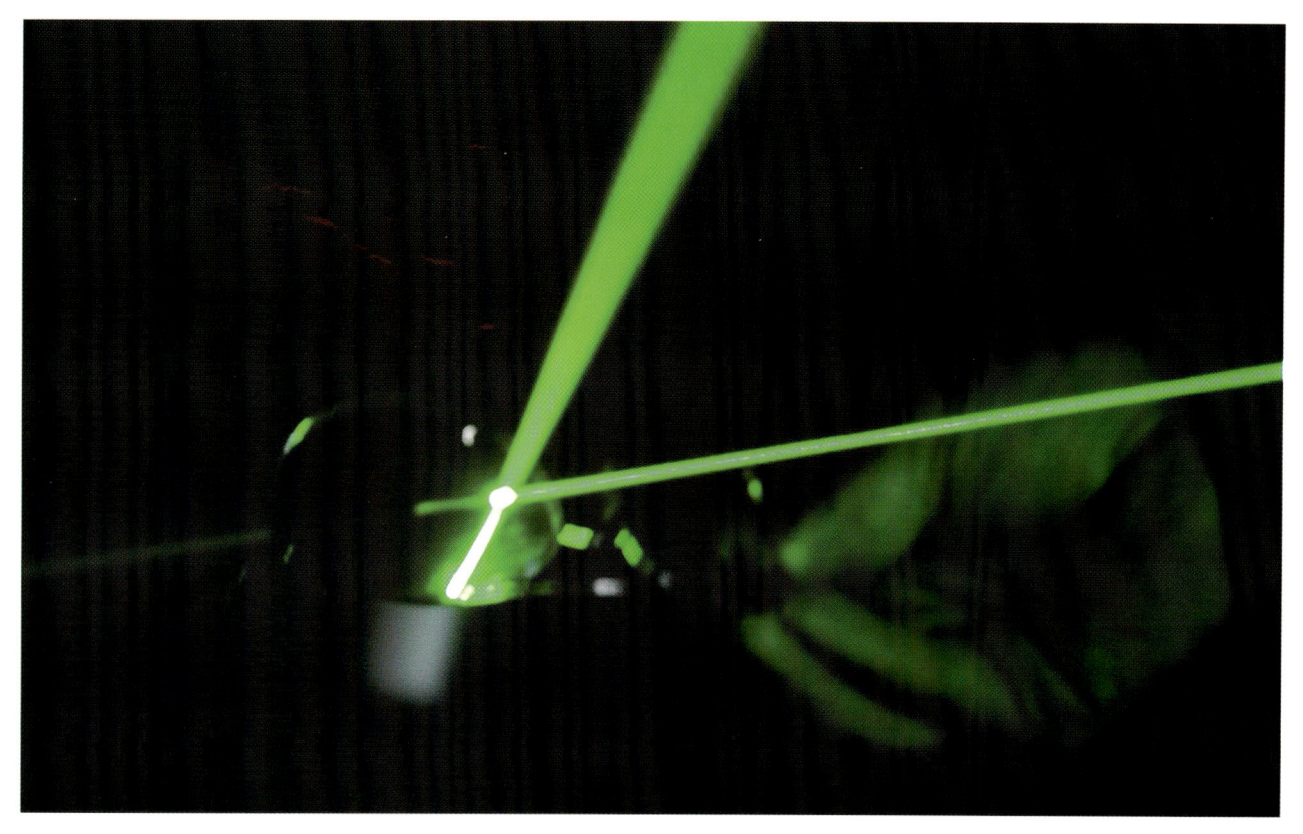

Once upon a time, lasers seemed like science fiction; nowadays, they play many roles in our everyday lives. They're found in everything from your CD player to a dentist's drill, from factories' metal-cutting machines to scientists' measuring tools, from supermarket scanners to a surgeon's tools.

Lasers

medical application as it cauterizes (burns) **blood vessels** at the very same time an incision is made. The benefit is less bleeding and infection. A cut with a traditional scalpel may cause profuse bleeding, while the same cut with a laser could produce nearly no bleeding at all. Some of the most common uses of lasers are in **LASIK** eye surgery, **tumor** and diseased-tissue removal, and **cosmetic surgery**.

ASK THE DOCTOR

In computer class, our teacher told us we shouldn't look at the red light on the bottom of the mouse because it's a laser. Is this true? Why can't we look at it?

A: Yes, that light is a laser, although it's not nearly as powerful as the type of laser used in things like surgery. Nevertheless, your teacher is right. You should never look directly at any laser, even a relatively weak one. Many of the lasers we use in daily life, like the laser on a laser mouse, are quite safe. There is a laser-safety rating system, and some of the lasers we use daily receive the safest classification: Class I "eye-safe." Nevertheless, it is always good to use caution. Not all the lasers we come in contact with on a daily basis are Class I. Many do have the potential to quickly burn certain parts of the eye, causing permanent damage. So the best course of action is to avoid looking directly at any laser.

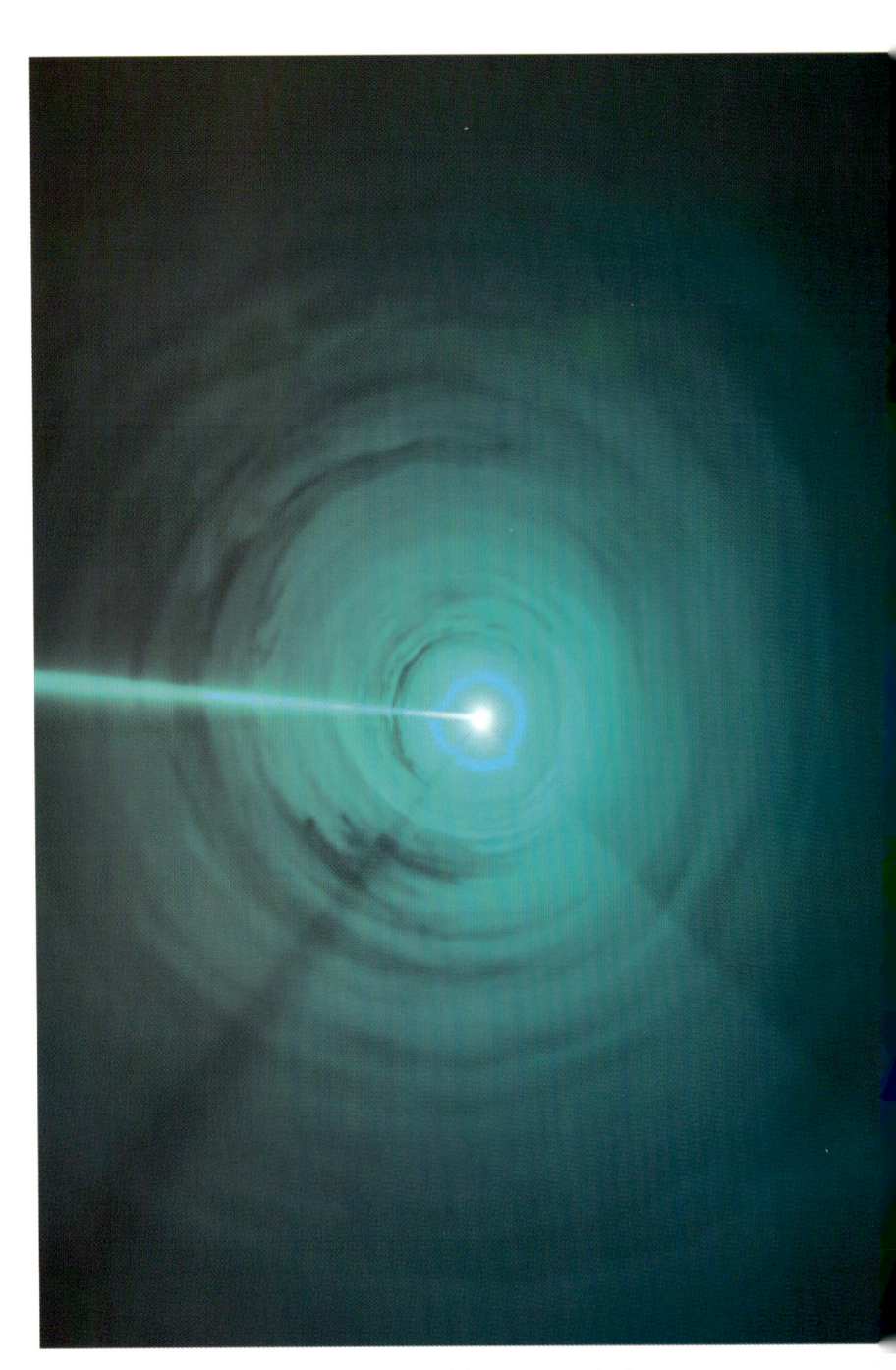

Unlike a normal flashlight, a typical laser emits light in an extremely narrow beam made up of synchronized light waves of a single color.

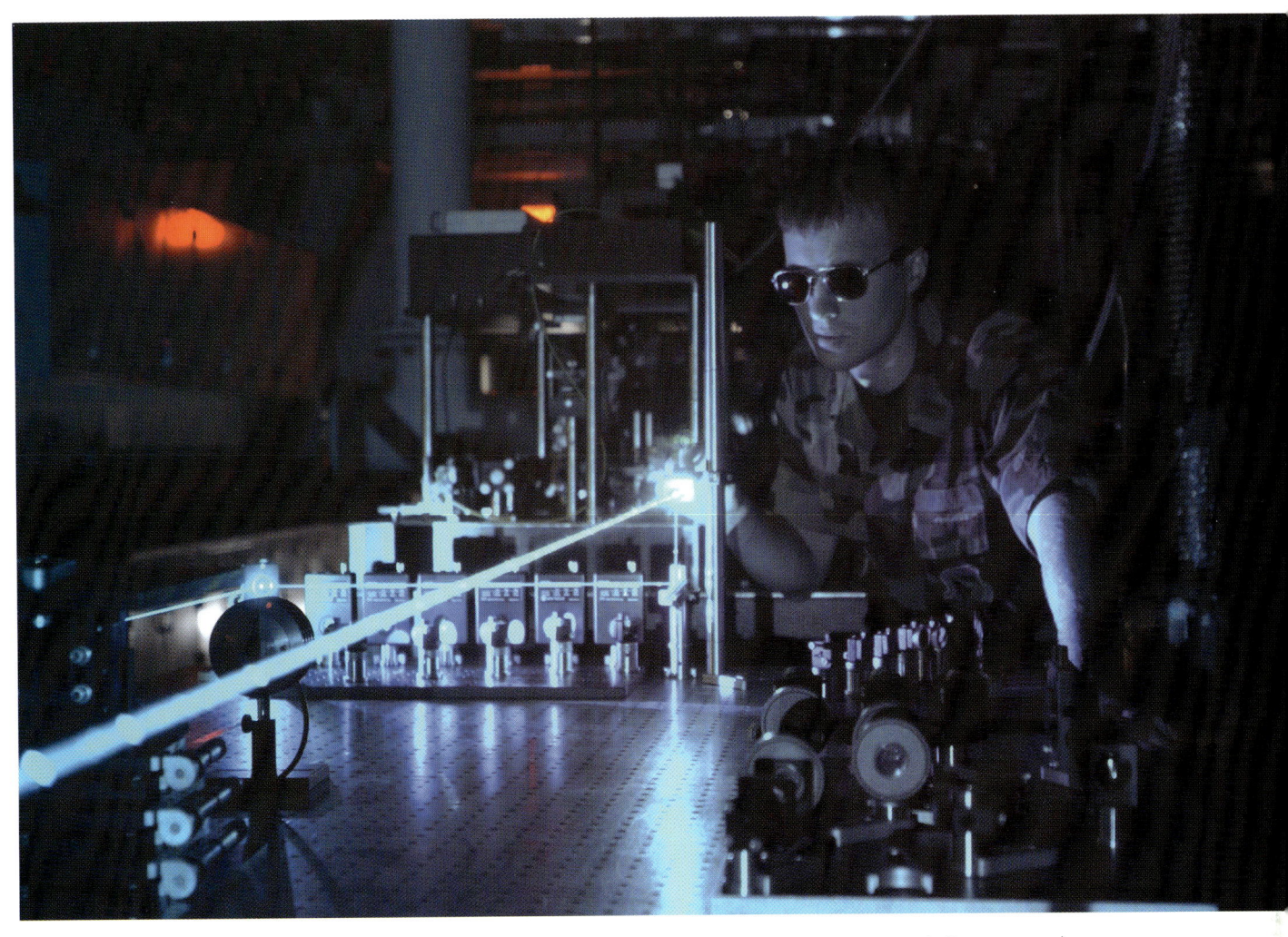

Scientists in both the military and the private sector are continuing to experiment with lasers, seeking new uses for this powerful tool.

LASIK SURGERY

LASIK stands for "laser-assisted *in situ* keratomileusis." It is laser surgery on the **eye** for the purpose of correcting vision that is impaired by nearsightedness, farsightedness, or astigmatism. LASIK surgery uses a laser to cut and shape the **cornea** (the clear covering on the front of the eye). The goal of the surgery is to reshape the cornea in such a way that will properly focus light into the eye, thus correcting certain types of vision problems. Many people who undergo LASIK surgery no longer need glasses or corrective lenses of any kind. LASIK surgery, however, is not without risks or problems, and since its start in 1990, a number of other laser-eye surgeries have been developed in an attempt to improve on LASIK surgery.

LAXATIVES

Laxatives are substances that encourage bowel movements. There are different types of laxatives, and they work in different ways. The gentlest laxatives are the naturally occurring fibers in plants. These add bulk and absorb water into the stool, causing it to pass

Laxatives

more quickly and easily through the intestines and out of the body. The best way to get enough dietary fiber is to eat a variety of plant foods every day. Legumes, whole grains, fruits, and vegetables all contain fiber. Some people boost the fiber in their daily diet with fiber supplements, often in the form of a powder that is mixed into liquid.

In addition to fiber, there are many other types of laxatives. Caffeine, for example, has a relatively strong laxative effect, and drinking a cup of coffee will result in an urge to have a bowel movement in many people. There are also many chemical laxatives. Laxatives can be powerful, and some chemical laxatives can be particularly harsh to the digestive system, causing irritation, frequent bowel movements, and in extreme cases, inability to control the bowels. These symptoms will subside once the laxative is out of the system. Strong chemical laxatives are used for some medical procedures. For example, a colonoscopy (an internal examination of the colon) requires that the bowels be completely evacuated of their contents prior to the start of the procedure. This is usually achieved with the use of a powerful chemical laxative.

Some people use laxatives under the mistaken belief that they will help them lose weight. This is false because laxatives work on the large intestine and the *colon*. Once food makes its way to the large intestine, most of the nutrients have already been absorbed. A laxative will help what remains pass out of the body faster, but they won't lead to a significant reduction in absorption to the body. Abuse of laxatives can be dangerous, leading to dehydration and improper nutrient absorption. Laxatives should never be used as a dieting device.

LEAD POISONING

Lead poisoning occurs when an unsafe amount of lead is ingested, inhaled, or otherwise taken into the body. Lead is extremely dangerous to humans, and even tiny amounts can cause permanent damage and disability.

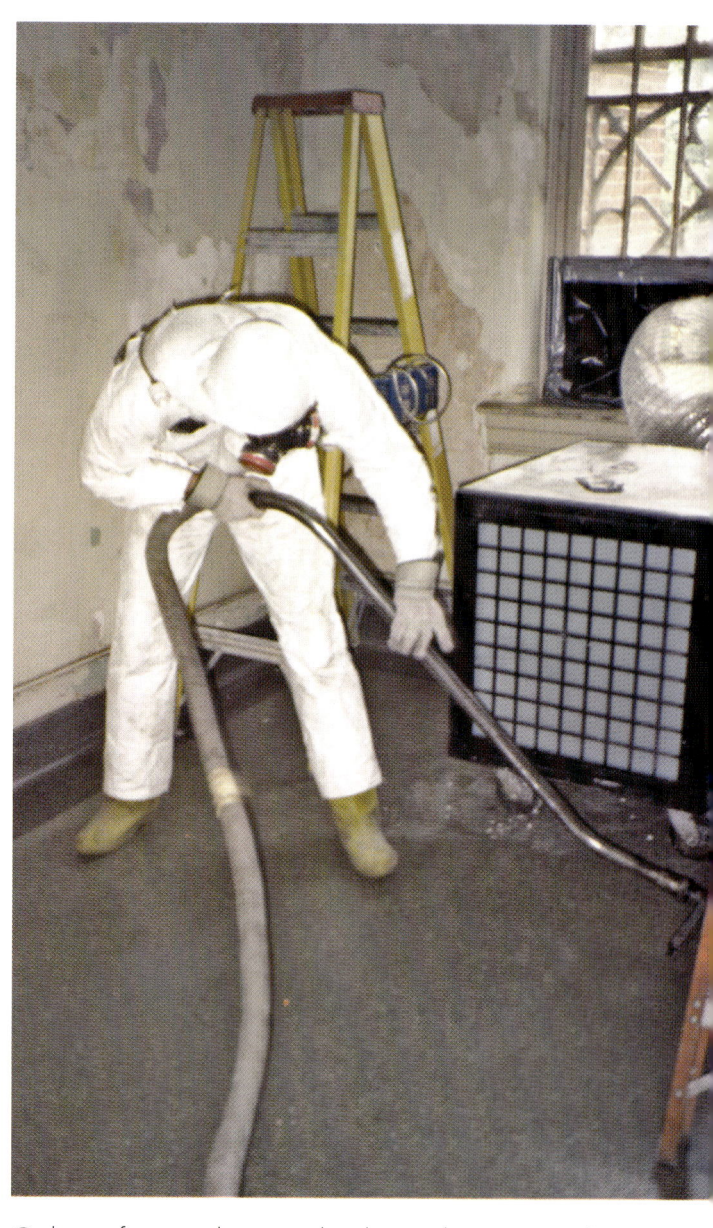

Only professionals trained in hazardous material removal should remove lead-based paint. These professionals must follow very detailed procedures to minimize, control, and contain the lead dust generated by the removal process.

Learning Disabilities

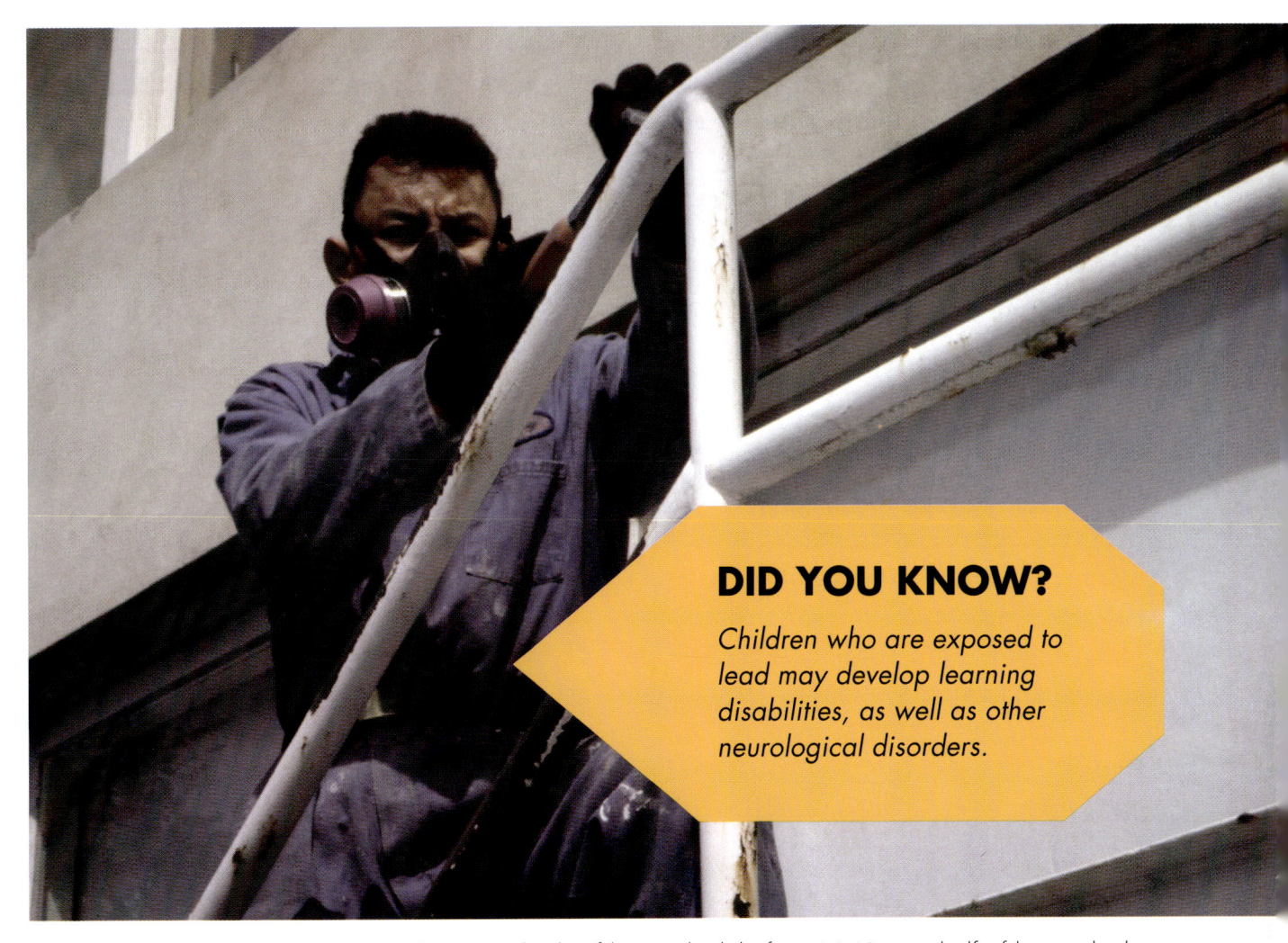

Heavily leaded paint was used in about two-thirds of homes built before 1940, one-half of homes built from 1940 to 1960, and some homes built after 1960. When removing old paint, workers should wear respirators designed to avoid inhaling lead.

DID YOU KNOW?
Children who are exposed to lead may develop learning disabilities, as well as other neurological disorders.

LEARNING DISABILITIES

Learning disabilities are a class of disabilities that inhibit a person's ability to take in, understand, or relay certain types of information. There are many types of learning disabilities, and some are quite common. Learning disabilities affect skills like reading, writing, listening, and speaking. They generally impact a person's functioning and success in school. They are not, however, related to intelligence.

Learning disabilities can be divided into four broad categories: input, integration, storage, and output. Input disabilities are those that affect a person's ability to take in information. Some people, for example, have difficulty with visual input, perhaps being unable to recognize shapes or sizes. Another example is when people have difficulty processing auditory information, perhaps being unable to screen out background noise in order to focus on important sounds, like a person speaking. Integration disabilities are those that relate to how the brain processes information once it has been taken in. For example, a person with an integration disability may be able to read a story but be unable

Learning Disabilities

to keep the events of the story arranged in proper sequence. A storage disability relates to memory and the ability to recall information. Finally, an output disability relates to an individual's ability to relay or communicate information. People communicate information in many ways, such as speaking, writing, gesturing, and drawing. An output disability impairs a person's ability to communicate in one or more of these ways.

A psychologist who administers achievement tests usually identifies learning disabilities through professional assessment. There is no "cure" for a learning disability. Treatment usual involves adjusting one's academic program to allow for presentation of information in the ways most compatible with the individual's abilities, structuring lessons in a way that allows more maximum information processing, and using evaluation techniques best-suited to the individual's output abilities. For example, if a person has difficulty processing written information, her lesson plans may be tailored to include more visual and auditory information. If a person has an output disability, he may be given more time to write tests or given tests in a different form (oral examinations rather than written examinations, for example). For some people, medication may also play a part in treatment of learning disabilities, particularly to improve concentration.

Dyslexia

Dyslexia is a learning disability that affects a person's functioning related to written language. Dyslexia most commonly results in problems with reading, writing, and spelling. A person with dyslexia struggles to process written information. This may manifest in a number of ways, including an inability to accurately determine what sounds individual letters make, distinguish properly between letters, or accurately spell words. Although dyslexia can greatly impair one's educational performance, it is not related to intelligence. A highly intelligent person with dyslexia may do poorly in school and get low grades because she cannot process the written material. If that same material were read to her, for example, she might be able to process it perfectly. Dyslexia often occurs along with other learning disabilities.

ASK THE DOCTOR

I just found out I have a learning disability—but my grandmother says if I'm patient, I'll outgrow it. Is that true?

A: No, unfortunately, learning disabilities are not something you can outgrow. If you have a learning disability, it's a permanent condition you'll have your entire life. However, now that your teachers and the other adults in your life know you have this condition, they can help you learn ways to cope with it. As you grow older, these coping techniques will become more automatic for you, so that your learning disability may not get in your way as much as it does now.

LEUKEMIA

Leukemia is a type of **cancer** that begins in **blood**-forming tissue such as bone **marrow**; this results in an abnormally high production and release of blood cells. Leukemia is a part of the group of cancers known as hematologic malignancies, or cancers of the blood system. Other hematologic malignancies include lymphoma and myeloma.

Leukemia is a general term, which encompasses many different cancer types:

- acute myelogenous leukemia (AML)
- acute lymphocytic leukemia (ALL)
- chronic myelogenous leukemia (CML)
- chronic lymphocytic leukemia (CLL)
- hairy cell leukemia
- large granular lymphocytic leukemia
- prolymphocytic leukemia
- T-cell chronic leukemia.

Abnormal Proliferation of Cells in Bone Marrow

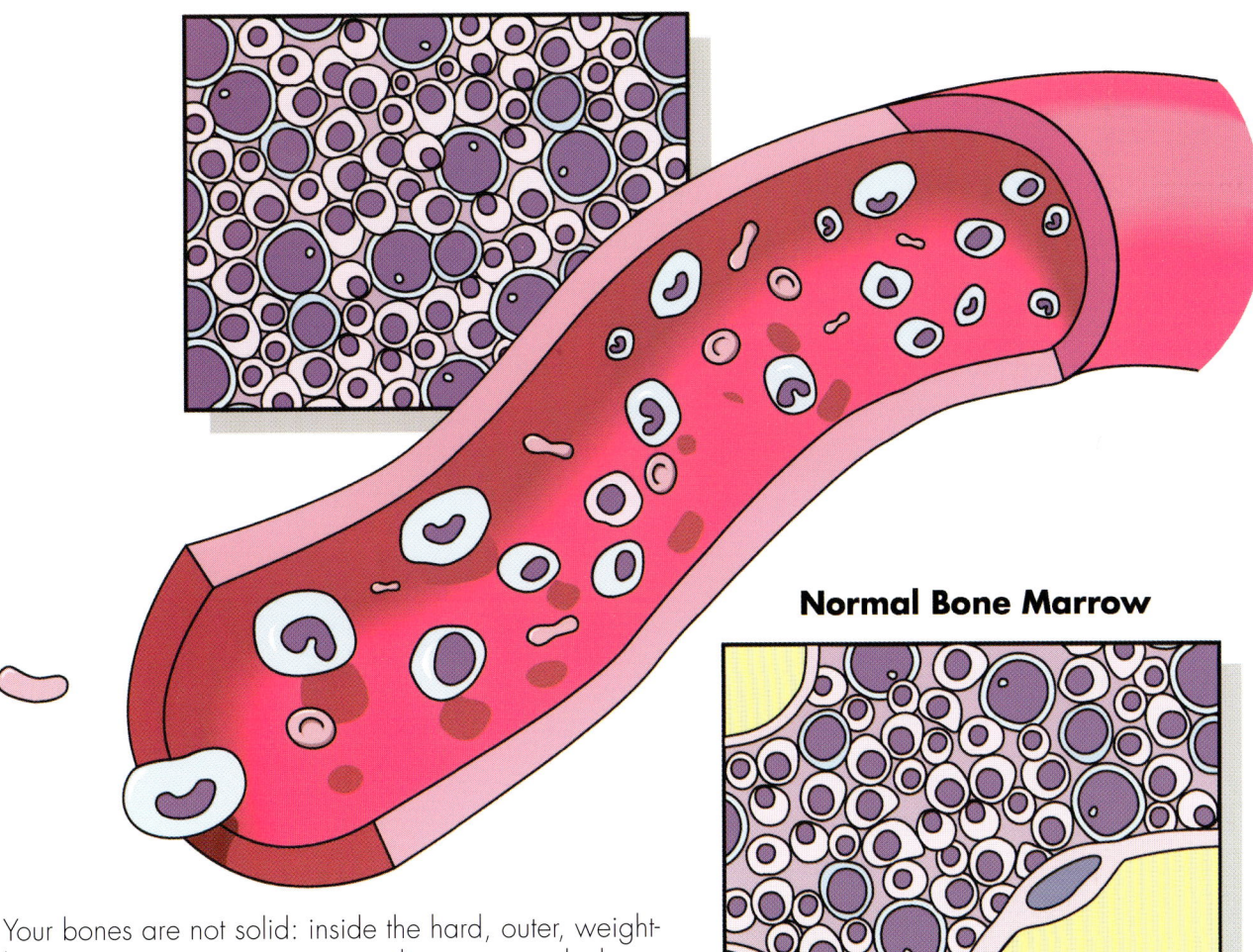

Normal Bone Marrow

Your bones are not solid: inside the hard, outer, weight-bearing area is an inner region, the marrow, which is one of the largest organs of the body. This is where many of your blood cells are created—but leukemia affects the normal production of blood cells within your bone marrow.

Leukemia

Acute leukemia results when the cancer results in rapid proliferation of immature blood cells. The crowd of immature cells means that the bone marrow is unable to produce healthy blood cells. Children and young adults are the most common population affected by acute leukemia, which must be treated immediately to halt the accumulation of malignant cells.

Chronic leukemia is the build-up of mature, though abnormal, blood cells. The chronic form progresses more slowly than the acute form, and usually occurs in older individuals.

Myelogenous refers to a change that takes place in a type of marrow cell that goes on to form red blood cells, some white blood cells or platelets. Lymphocyctic, on the other hand, indicates that the cancerous change occurs in a type of marrow cell that forms lymphocytes (white blood cells that are a part of the immune system).

Causes

For most types of leukemia, the causes and risk factors are not well understood. Some risk factors, such as exposure to high levels of radiation, have been identified. However, most people who have the specific risk factors do not get leukemia, and most people who do get leukemia do not have any of these risk factors.

DID YOU KNOW?

Each year, about 30,000 new cases of leukemia are diagnosed. It accounts for about one-third of all cancers in children younger than 15, and it causes an estimated 22,000 deaths each year. It is the sixth leading cause of cancer deaths among men and the seventh leading cause of cancer deaths among women.

ASK THE DOCTOR

My sister has leukemia. One of my friends told me that my sister made herself get sick because she's the type of person who worries all the time. My sister is really scared now because she's afraid she's going to die. If she doesn't stop worrying, will it keep her from getting better?

A: Your sister did not make herself get sick by worrying. And it's normal for her to feel scared now. Although our minds and our bodies are connected, researchers have found nothing to indicate that people can make themselves get better simply by thinking positive thoughts. Relaxation techniques, meditation, and prayer, however, have all been shown to improve patients' peace of mind, so you might encourage your sister to try one of these when she feels scared—and you might find it helpful too!

Leukemia

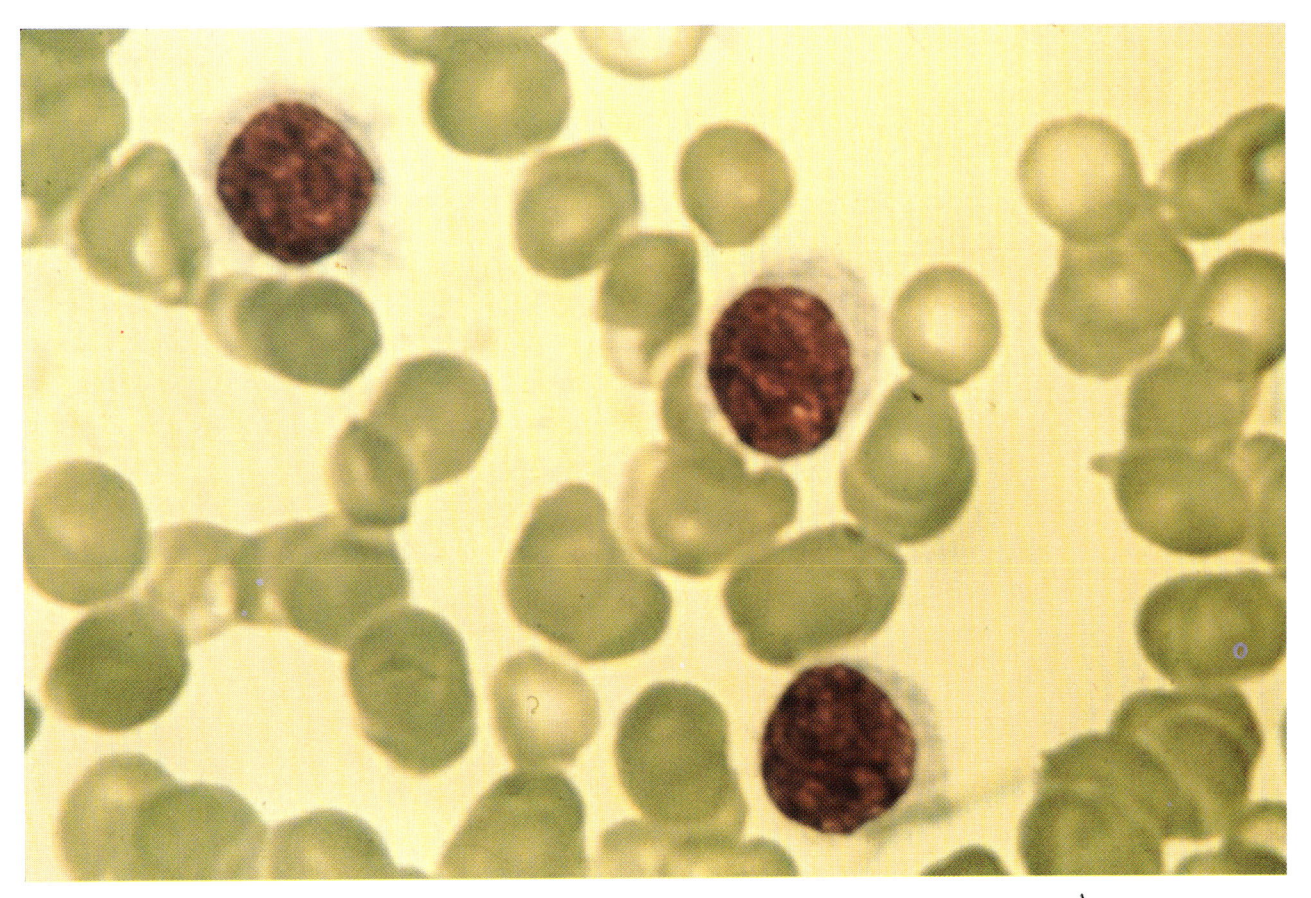

This magnified slide of a patient's blood shows too many white blood cells, indicating that this person may have leukemia.

Some risk factors that have been identified for AML include:

- chronic exposure to benzene levels that exceed federally approved safety limits
- radiation and chemotherapies used in treatment of another cancer
- exposure to tobacco smoke
- Down syndrome and other genetic disorders

Symptoms

Symptoms of leukemia vary depending on the specific type, but can be similar to other common ailments. Chronic leukemia may not cause any symptoms, so that some people only get the diagnosis after a routine blood test. Others may notice enlarged lymph nodes, lethargy, shortness of breath, or an increase in infections.

For acute leukemia, symptoms include:

- lethargy
- shortness of breath
- pale skin
- fever
- slow healing of skin wounds
- unexplained bruising
- small red spots under the skin
- bone and joint aches
- low white blood cell count

Leukemia

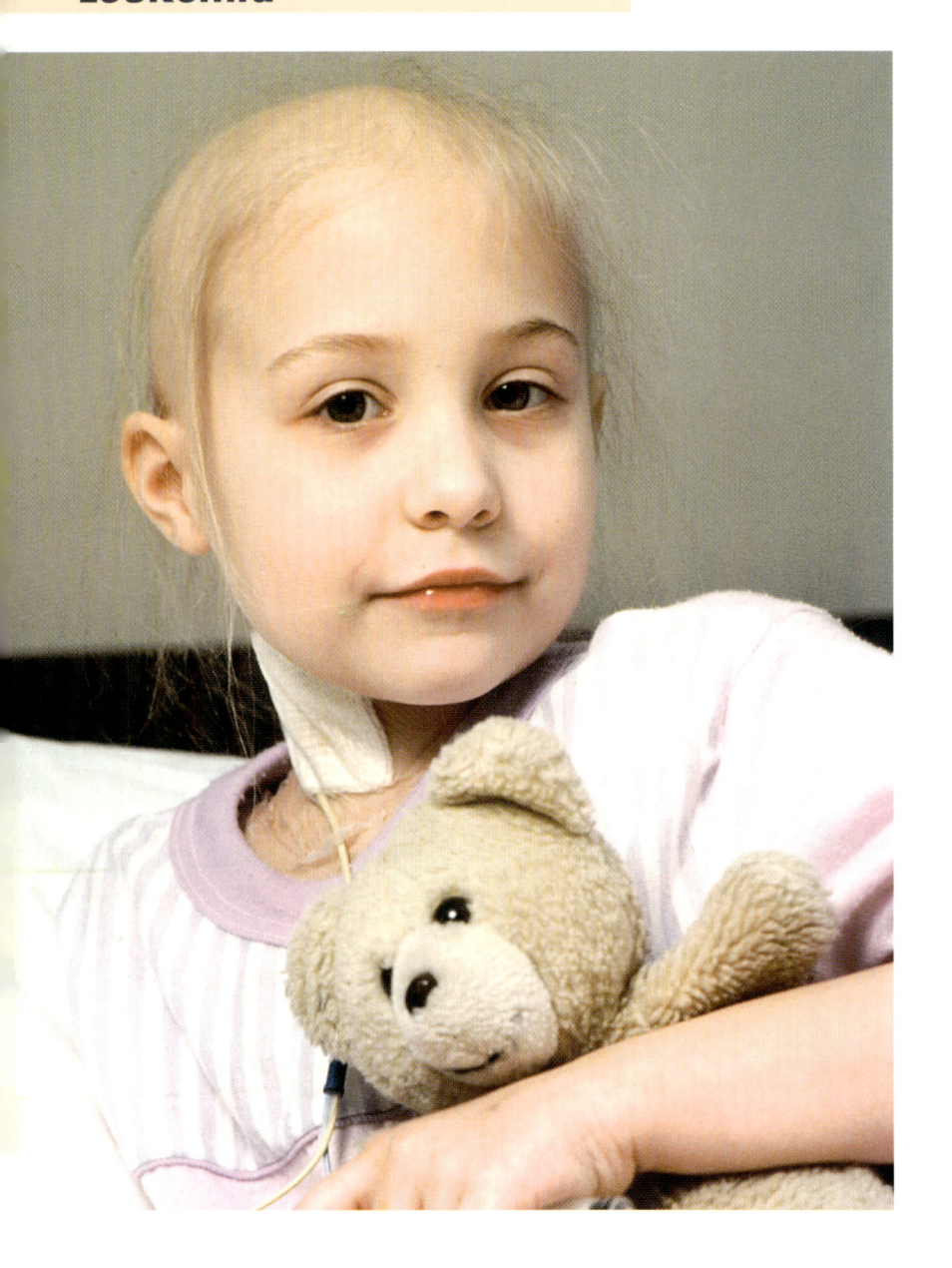

> ### ASK THE DOCTOR
> **Why do cancer patients always lose their hair?**
>
> **A:** Cancer patients do not always lose their hair. It is however, a common side effect of both chemotherapy and radiation therapy. Both of these forms of treatment damage and kill healthy cells along with the cancer cells they target. The death of the healthy cells is what causes the unpleasant side effects of treatment, including nausea, vomiting, fatigue, and hair loss. Usually the hair loss is temporary; the hair will grow back once treatments are stopped. However, radiation therapy can sometimes cause permanent hair loss.

Hair loss can be a difficult side effect to cope with—but it is almost always temporary.

Since none of these symptoms are unique to leukemia, special blood and bone marrow tests are necessary to make an accurate diagnosis. If leukemia is suspected, a doctor will take a complete blood count (CBC), which measures the levels of each type of blood cells. A biopsy of the bone marrow may also be used to identify the leukemia cell-type.

Treatment

Treatment for leukemia is complex—you can't just remove the source of the problem, because the body needs bone marrow to produce blood cells. The treatment will vary depending on the type of leukemia, as well as the patient's age and general health. There are a number of therapies used, including chemotherapy, radiation therapy, bone marrow transplant, and biological therapy.

Chemotherapy

Chemotherapy uses chemicals, or drugs, to kill cancer cells. The drugs are injected into a vein with a needle, or may be swallowed. Chemotherapy kills cancer cells, but

Leukemia

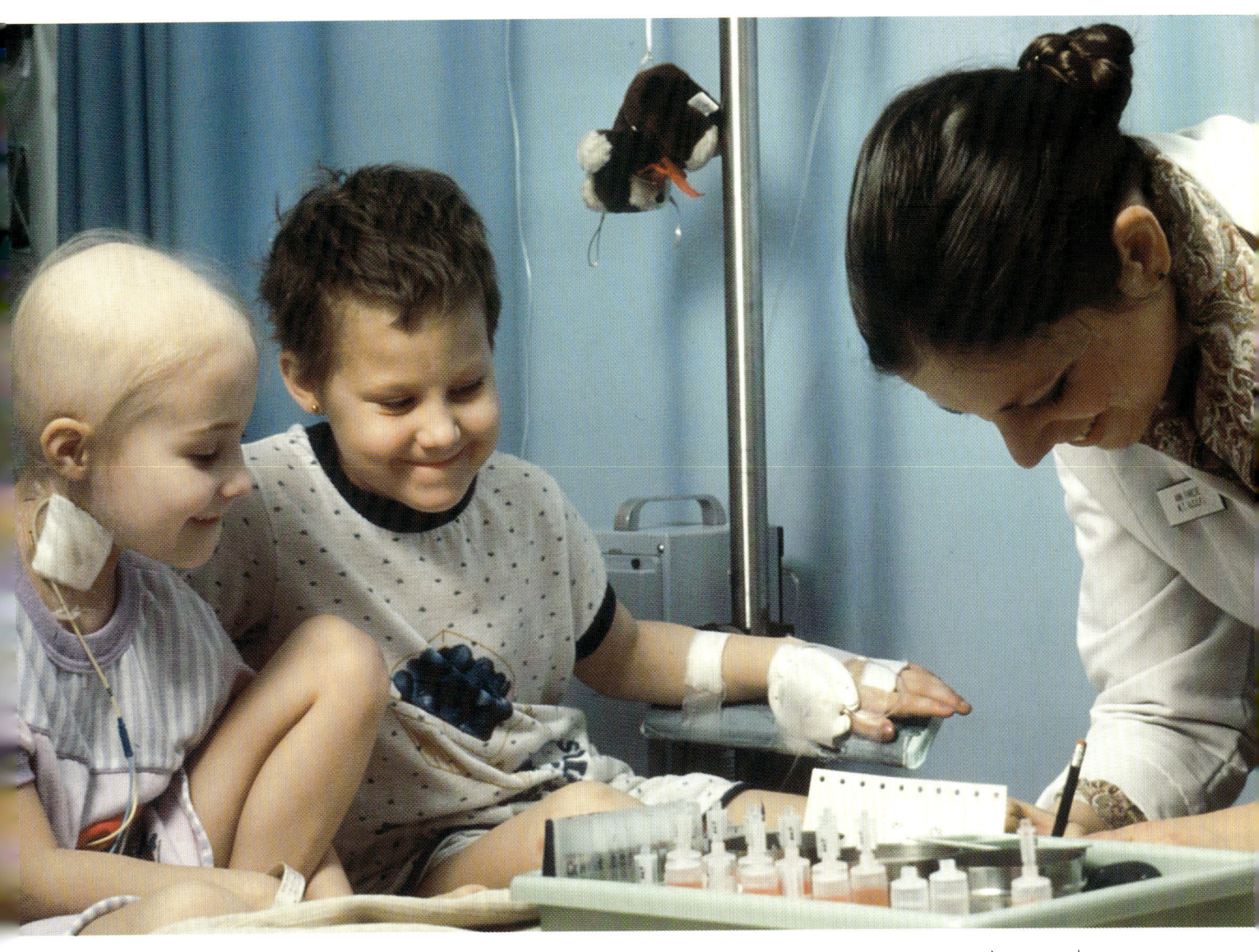

Leukemia affects many children around the world; in some countries, it is more common than in others. Luckily, however, with treatment, most children with leukemia will live normal lives free from the disease.

because the chemicals travel throughout the body in the bloodstream, they also kill healthy cells.

Radiation Therapy

Radiation therapy uses X-rays, or other high-energy radiation to damage cancer cells and stop their growth. The radiation may be directed at a specific part of the body, or it may be directed at the entire body. Either way, healthy cells may be damaged along with the cancer cells.

Bone Marrow Transplant

A bone marrow transplant replaces the cancerous marrow with healthy marrow given by a compatible donor. The first step of this treatment is to destroy all the cancerous marrow using either radiation or chemotherapy. Sometimes, when a patient is in remission, she may save some of her healthy bone marrow for use if the cancer returns in the future. The saved marrow can then be used for something called an autologous transplant

Leukemia

because it is the patient's own marrow being returned to her body.

Stem cell transplant is similar to bone marrow transplant, except the transplanted cells are stem cells collected from the bloodstream instead of the bone marrow. This procedure is often preferred because recovery time is shorter, and the risk of infection is lower than with a bone marrow transplant.

Biological Therapy

Biological therapy is also called immunotherapy, because it uses substances that increase the immune system's response to cancer. This type of therapy is also used in combination with chemotherapy or radiation therapy to help fight the side effects of these treatments.

Type-Specific Treatments

Specialized treatments for specific types of leukemia include kinase inhibitors, which are often the first line of defense for patients with CML. Promyelocytic leukemia, a subtype of AML, is sometimes treated using arsenic trioxide and all-trans retinoic acid (ATRA) in combination with other chemotherapy drugs. These drugs target cancer cells with a specific gene mutation. Clinical trials are also an option for patients who want experimental therapies or new combinations of accepted therapies.

Remission

The goal of any cancer treatment is to bring the patient into remission. After a regimen of treatment has been completed, the doctor will re-run the test used to diagnose the cancer initially. If no cancer is found, the patient is said to be in remission. Periodic retesting will be required to make sure the cancer does not come back. The longer the individual stays cancer-free, the fewer bone marrow tests will be necessary.

Life with Leukemia

A diagnosis of leukemia is scary for the patient and his family, but many people survive the diagnosis and lead happy, healthy lives. One of the most important parts of the healing process for both the patient and his family is to have a strong support system. Whether the support comes from family, friends, or a formal group, it is vital to have a place to talk about your feelings and concerns. A support group is also a good place to learn more about leukemia; educating yourself about the illness and treatment will help you know what to expect. Finally, eating well, getting enough sleep, and staying active are all important while dealing with the stress and fatigue of cancer treatments. Some days will be harder than others, but stay motivated, set reasonable goals, and maintain your normal activities as much as possible.

For more information, visit the Leukemia & Lymphoma Society at: www.leukemia-lymphoma.org/all_page.adp?item_id=7026#leukemia

DID YOU KNOW?

Most cases of leukemia occur in older adults; more than half of all cases occur after age 67.

Life Expectancy

LIFE EXPECTANCY

Life expectancy is the number of years a person is expected to live based on factors including sex, date of birth, country of birth or residence, and race or ethnicity. Life expectancies are averages based on calculations of the number of years lived by members of a given category.

In general, life expectancies worldwide today are much higher than at previous times in human history, although there is still great variation and discrepancy in life expectancies depending on where a person is born or lives. According to the CIA World Factbook, average life expectancy for people living in the United States is approximately 75 years for men and 81 years for women. Canada has a higher life expectancy: approximately 77 years for men and approximately 84 years for women. The country

Life expectancy 1950-2005

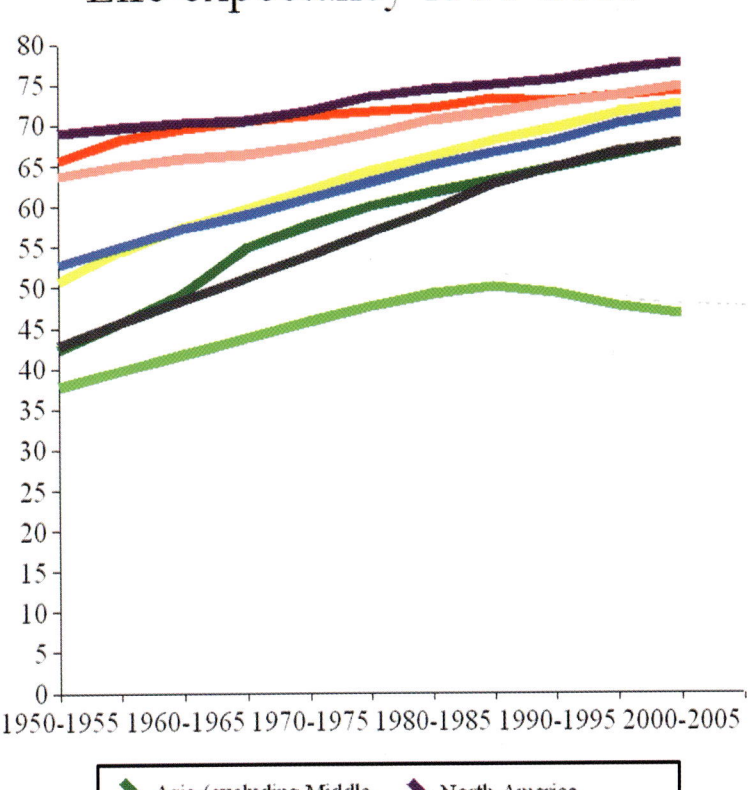

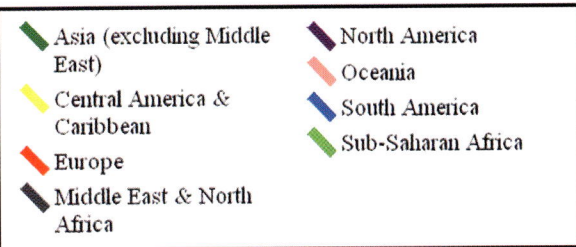

Legend:
- Asia (excluding Middle East)
- Central America & Caribbean
- Europe
- Middle East & North Africa
- North America
- Oceania
- South America
- Sub-Saharan Africa

ASK THE DOCTOR

People always say that men don't live as long as women. Why?

A: That is a difficult question to answer. Certainly not all men have shorter lives than women, but when averaged out over entire populations, women do tend to live a number of years longer than men. There are probably many factors resulting in this situation. For example, more men die in accidents, homicides, and suicides than women. Men tend to smoke at a higher rate than women, which would lead to more smoking-related diseases and health complications in men. Some theorists have also posited that men have traditionally held higher-stress jobs than women, leading to increased negative health effects in men. And of course, there are also physiological differences between the bodies of men and women, leading to differences in how they age. But how large a role these differences play in life expectancy is hotly debated. You may find it interesting to know, however, that it is only fairly recently that women have surpassed men in life expectancy. In the past, so many women died during childbirth that their overall life expectancy was less than men's.

Life Expectancy

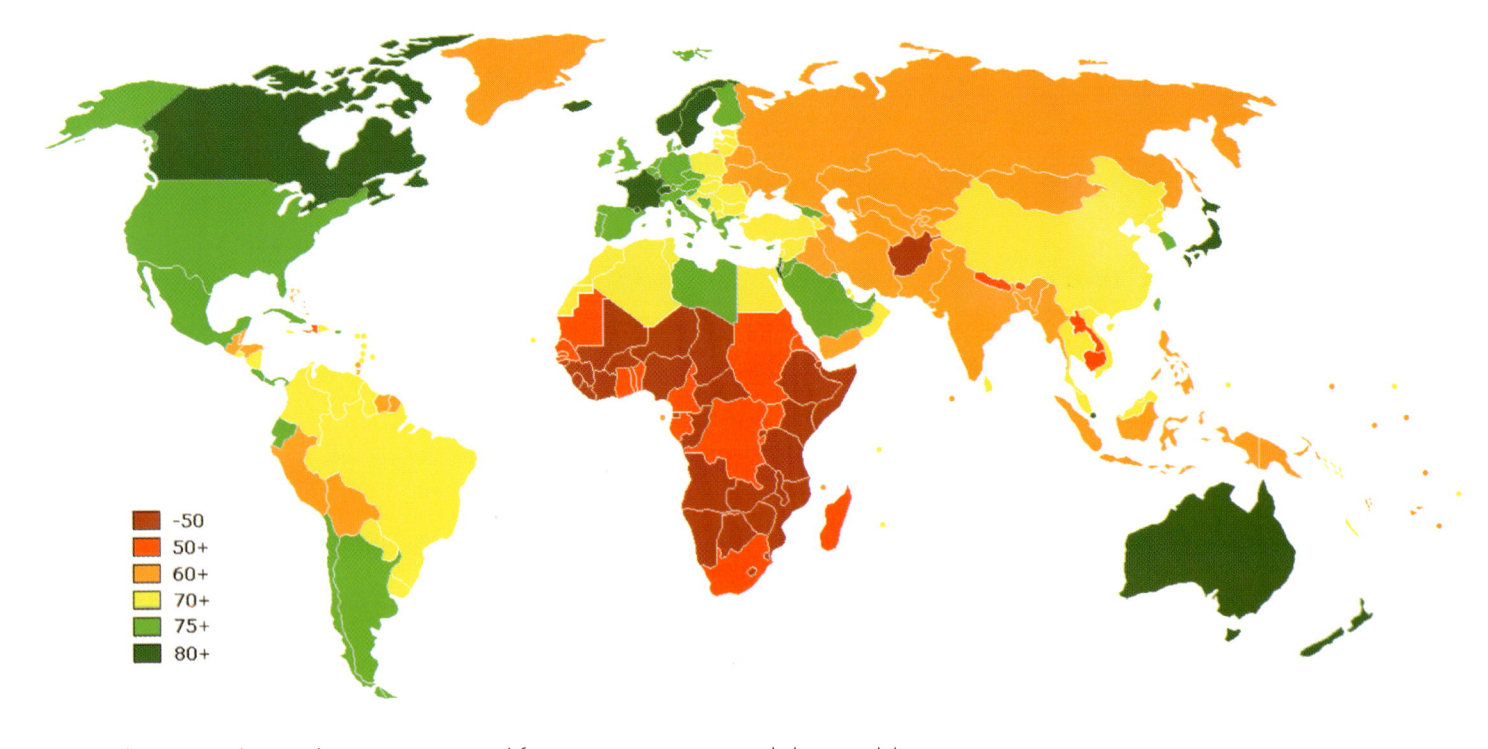

This map shows the variations in life expectancy around the world.

with the highest life expectancy is Andorra, with approximately 81 years for men and 87 years for women. The country with the lowest life expectancy is Swaziland with an average of approximately 32 years for men and 33 years for women. Worldwide, the average life expectancy is approximately 64 years for men and 68 years for women.

LIGAMENTS

Ligaments are sinewy tissues that attach bones to each other. This type of ligament is also sometimes called an articular ligament. They play a key role in the body's *joints*

Ligaments hold together the bones in your ankle (above) and in your spine (next page).

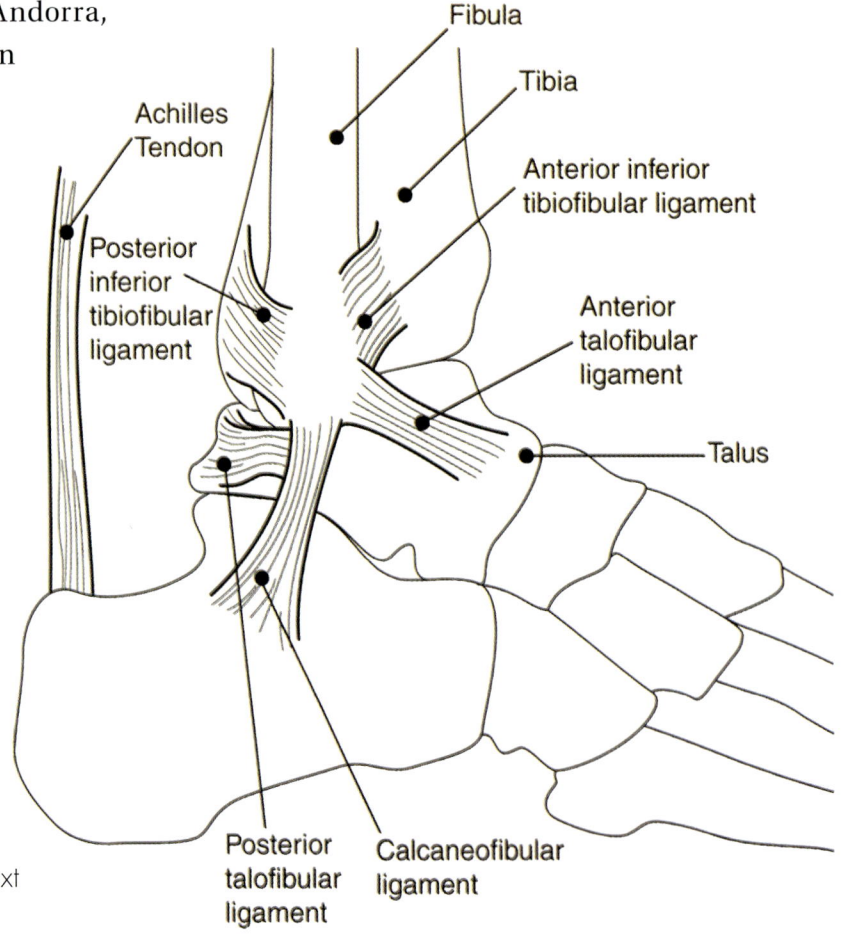

64

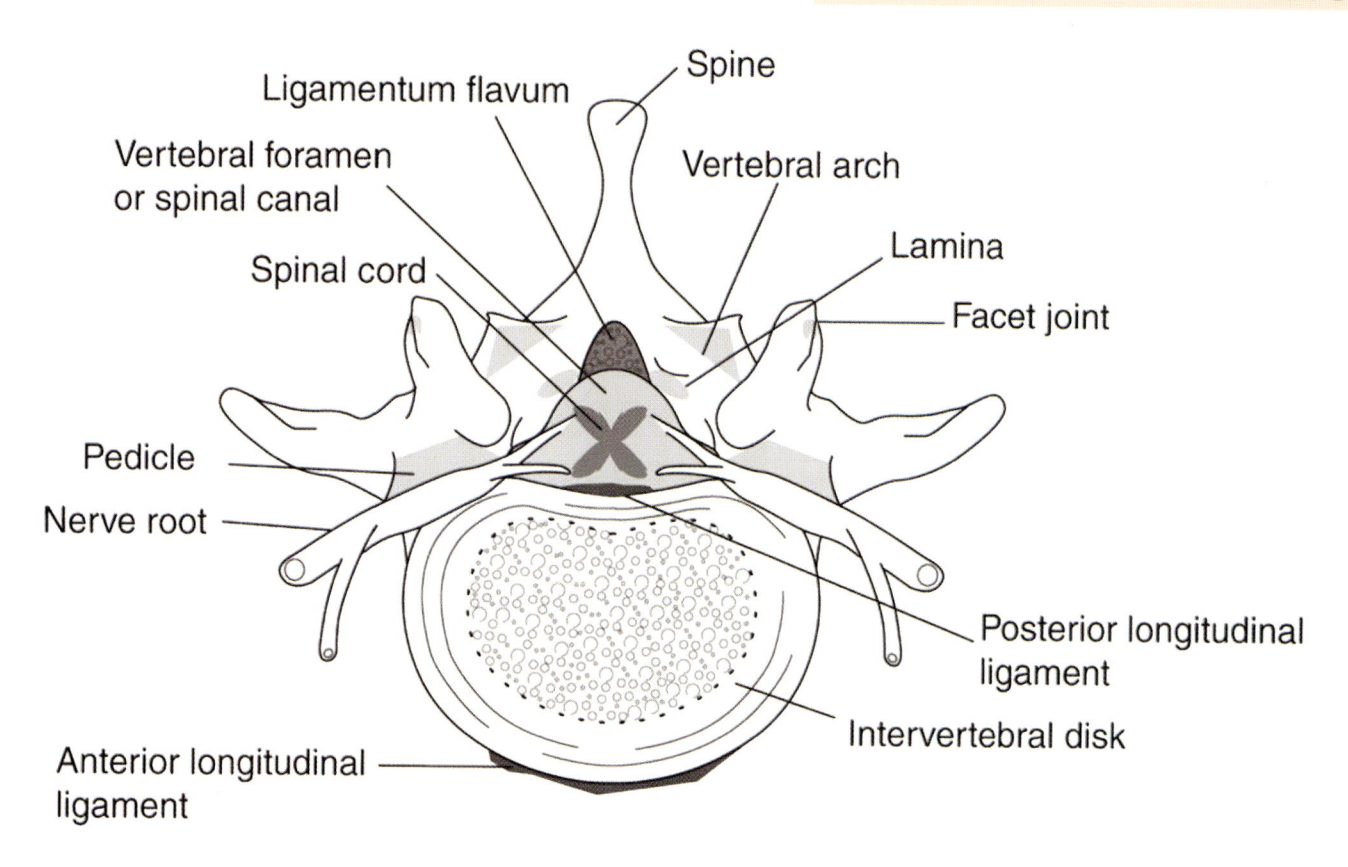

Structures of the Spine

by holding bones together, supporting or reinforcing the joint structure, and restricting mobility to the type of movement for which the joint is designed.

Ligaments are made mostly of a tissue called **collagen**. Although they are tough and fibrous, they do have a certain amount of elasticity, allowing them to bend and stretch. The more elastic a person's ligaments are, the more flexibility they will show at the joints. This can be beneficial in certain sports and performing arts, but too much elasticity can also make an individual more prone to certain types of injury. In injury, ligaments are sometimes stretched enough to cause permanent weakening of the joint. Weakened ligaments make the joint more susceptible to dislocation. Stretched or torn ligaments are sometimes corrected using surgery.

LIPOSUCTION

Liposuction is an elective cosmetic procedure for removing **fat** from the body.

LIVER

The liver is a vital organ that plays a key role in a number of important processes in the body. It is the body's largest **gland** (a gland is an organ that creates a substance and secretes it into the body), and it is essential for certain metabolic functions. Liver processes include storing a simple sugar called glycogen for energy, destroying old or extra red blood cells, creating certain types of proteins, cleansing the body of certain wastes and toxins, and creating and excreting **bile**, a compound that plays an important role in

Liver

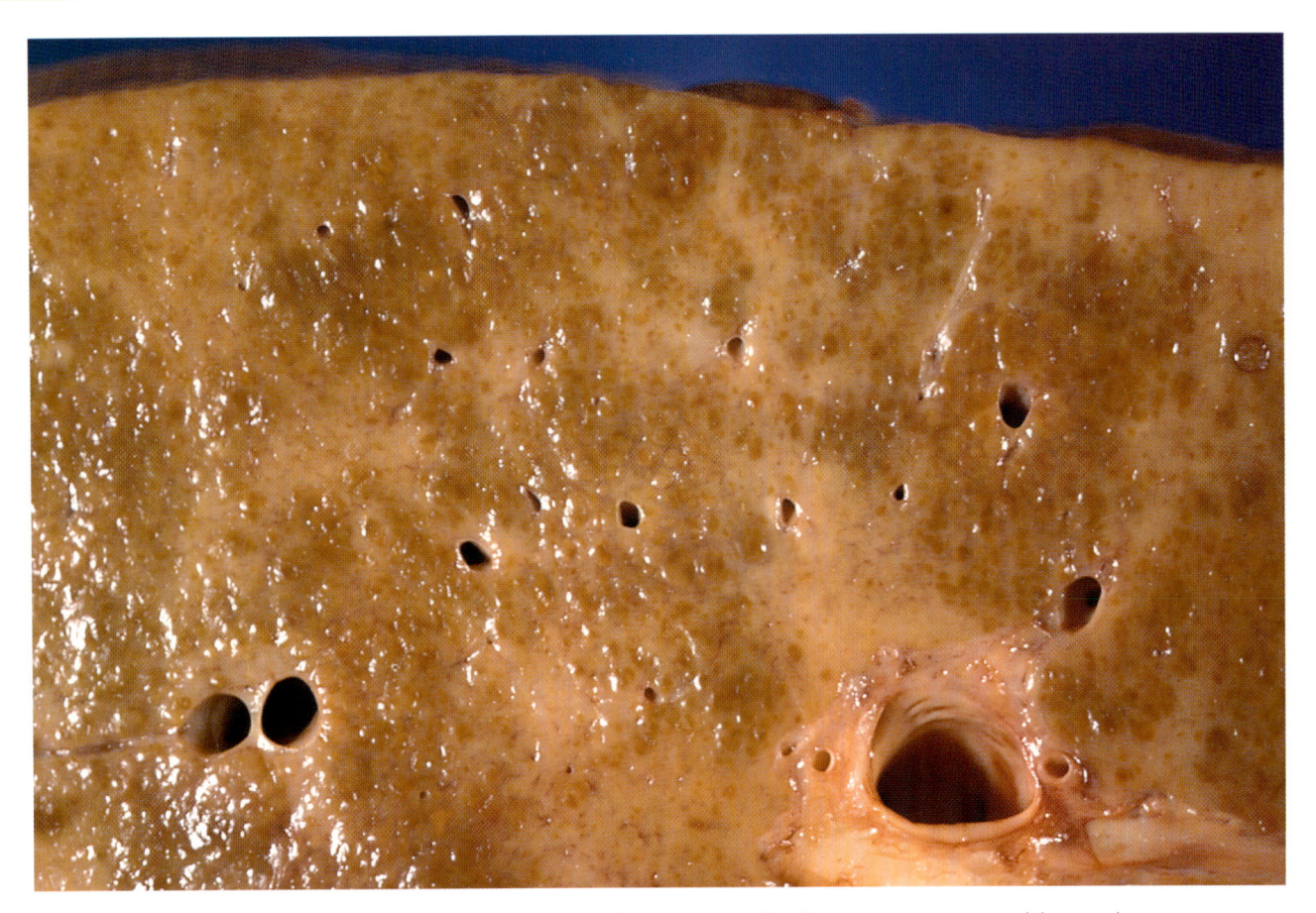

This liver specimen is unnaturally pale, due to a dense network of scar tissue caused by cirrhosis in response to chronic injury from alcohol abuse.

digestion. Conditions and diseases of the liver can be extremely serious, as a functional liver is essential for life. The liver does, however, have a great capacity for repair and regeneration and can heal from certain types of damage. Liver transplants are one of the more common forms of organ transplant.

Bile

Bile is an alkaline substance, meaning it has a high pH (greater than 7) and can neutralize acids. Bile is created in and secreted by the liver and stored in the **gallbladder** between meals. On its way to the gallbladder, bile passes through a number of ducts. When digestion is taking place, bile is released from the gallbladder into the first section of the small intestine. Here, it helps to complete the digestive process that began in the **stomach**.

Cirrhosis

Cirrhosis is the replacement of healthy liver tissue with scar tissue. This usually happens as a result of extensive disease of the liver or damage to the liver by substances like alcohol. It is very dangerous, as the scar tissue hardens the liver and impedes the liver's function. Once cirrhosis occurs, it cannot be reversed. If the cirrhosis is not extensive, lifestyle changes or treatment of disease may be able to prevent the condition from worsen-

Liver

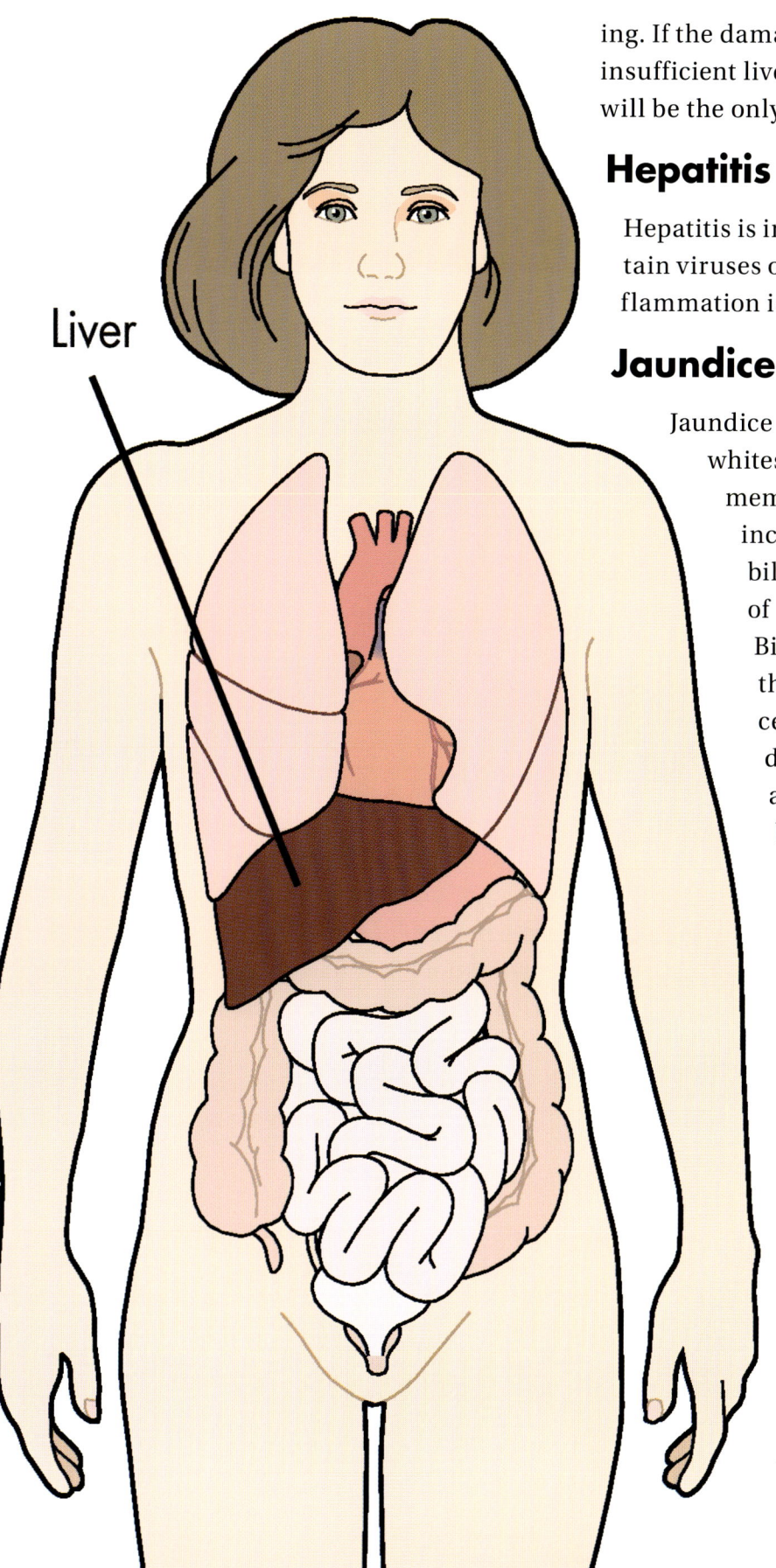

ing. If the damage is extensive and results in insufficient liver function, a liver transplant will be the only option to sustain life.

Hepatitis

Hepatitis is inflammation of the liver. Certain viruses often cause it, but any liver inflammation is considered hepatitis.

Jaundice

Jaundice is yellowing of the skin, whites of the eyes, and mucous membranes. It is caused by an increase of a chemical called bilirubin, and it can be a sign of serious liver malfunction. Bilirubin is the by-product of the destruction of red blood cells in the body. The regular destruction of red blood cells and eventual metabolism of bilirubin is a normal daily function of the body, but jaundice can occur when something goes wrong with this process.

A number of things can cause jaundice, and the causes are divided into three overall categories: pre-hepatic, hepatic, and post-hepatic. Pre-hepatic jaundice occurs when red blood cells are being destroyed at a higher-than-normal rate in the body, resulting in a flood of bilirubin. Hepatic jaundice occurs when liver malfunction prevents the proper metabolism of bilirubin. Hepatic

Liver

jaundice is extremely common in newborns because their livers are usually not completely functional at birth. This form of hepatic jaundice is called "neonatal" jaundice. In some cases, phototherapy to break down excess bilirubin may be necessary until the infant's liver is ready to perform this task on its own. The final form of jaundice is posthepatic jaundice, which occurs when something, usually gallstones, interrupts the flow of bile. Jaundice is a symptom, rather than a disease, so treatment relies on identification and successful treatment of the underlying cause.

For more information, visit the American Liver Foundation at: www.liverfoundation.org

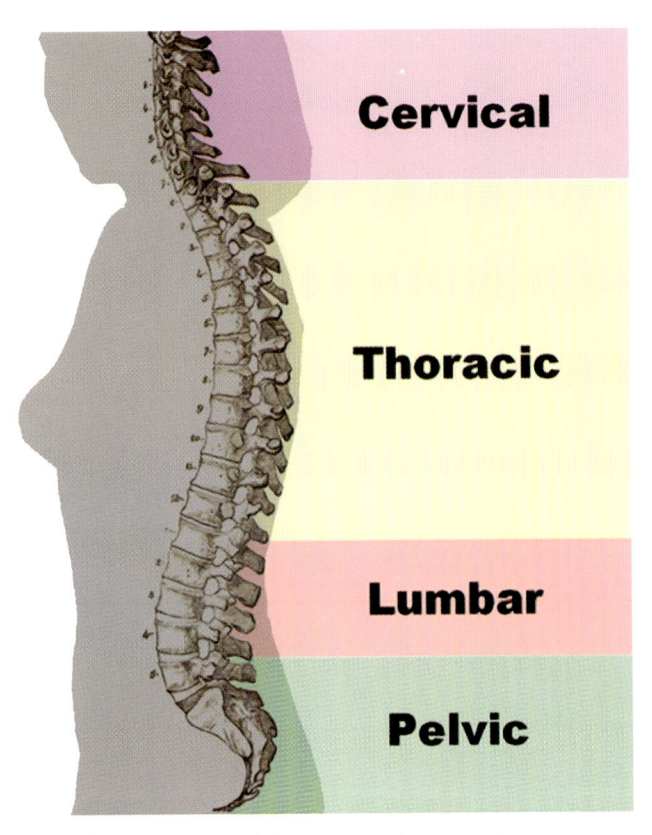

LOCAL ANESTHETICS

Local anesthetics are substances used to numb small areas or regions of the body.

LOWER-BACK PAIN

Low **back** pain, commonly called "lower-back pain," is musculoskeletal pain located in the lumbar region of the back. The lumbar is the portion of the body from the diaphragm to the pelvis. It is also often called the abdominal region. The lumbar spine is the portion of the spinal column in the lumbar region. Low back pain can be acute (sudden and temporary, such as from an injury) or chronic (long-lasting and/or recurring).

Accidents and injuries cause some of the most common forms of acute low back pain. Nevertheless, the pain may be quite long-lasting, as low back injuries can take a significant period of time to heal. Some of the most common causes of chronic low back pain are **rheumatoid arthritis**, **osteoarthritis**, or damage to the intervertebral discs. These causes usually develop gradually over time and can be much more difficult to treat since they involve significant structural damage in the affected area.

The four regions of the spine; low back pain affects the lumbar region.

DID YOU KNOW?

Nearly everyone at some point has back pain that interferes with daily life. North Americans spend more than $50 billion each year on low back pain; it is the most common cause of job-related disability.

Lower-Back Pain

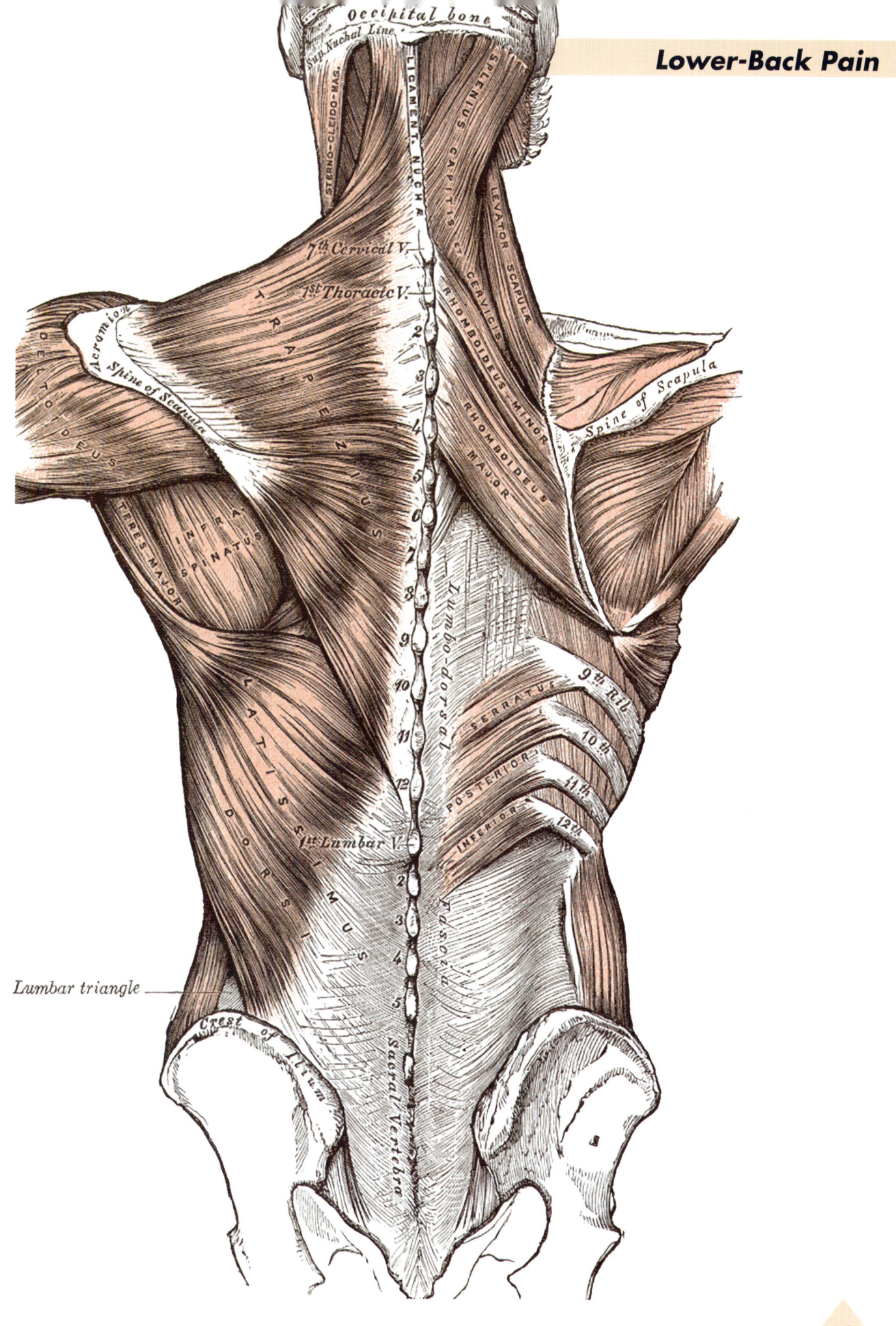

69

LSD

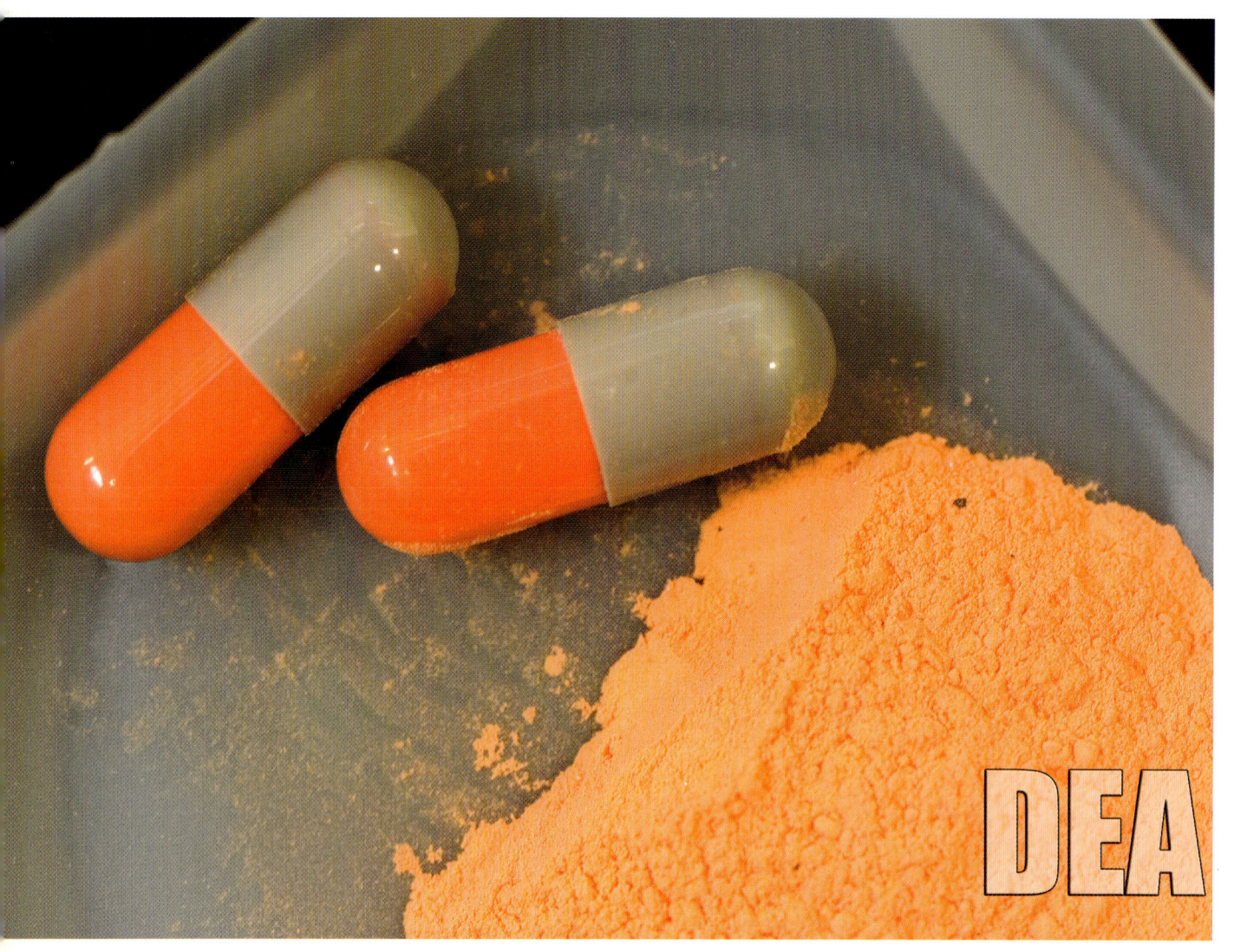

LSD comes in a variety of forms, including capsules.

LSD

Lysergic acid diethylamide (LSD) is a psychedelic or hallucinogenic drug. Hallucinogenic drugs cause distortions in a person's perception of reality, so that she sees things, hears sounds, and feels sensations that are not real. Sandoz Laboratories originally introduced LSD in 1938 as a therapeutic drug. Since 1966, however, it has been illegal in much of the world, with a Schedule I classification under the U.S. Controlled Substances Act.

Schedule I drugs:

- have a high potential for abuse
- have no currently accepted medical use
- are considered unsafe for use, even under medical supervision

The effects of LSD are different for each person, and even different for the same person depending on the amount taken, and the environment in which the drug is taken. Physical effects may include dilated

LSD

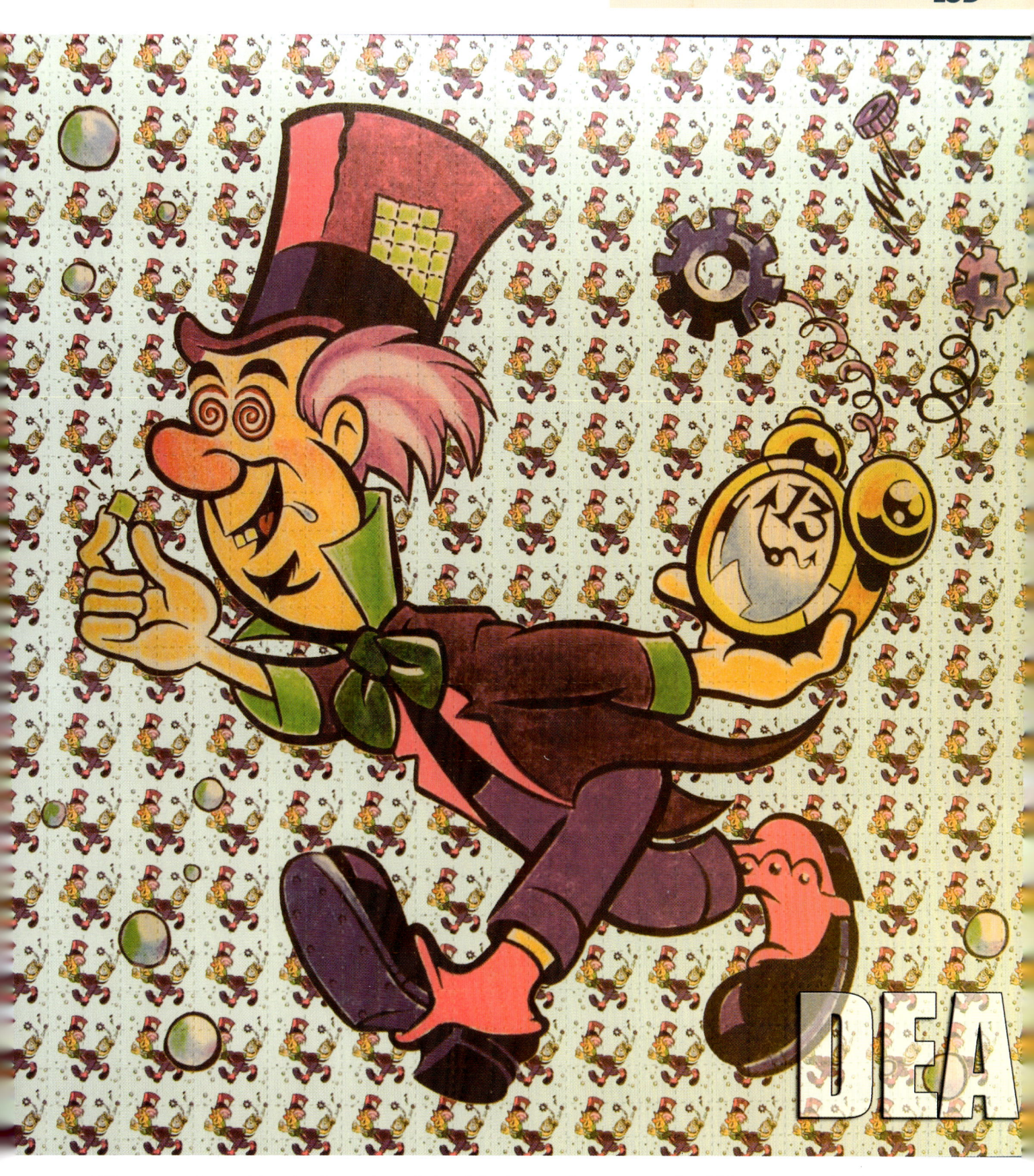

LSD is most often sold in the form of small, brightly designed squares made of blotter paper that has been dipped in LSD.

pupils, increased body temperature, increased heart rate and blood pressure, sweating, loss of appetite, dry mouth, and tremors. The psychological effects vary more than the physical effects. A person usually refers to his experience with LSD as a "trip," which will often last as many as 12 hours. A "bad trip" occurs when the **hallucinations** are scary or depressing. LSD is not considered addictive, as it does not produce compulsive drug-seeking behavior. However, tolerance to the drug does increase with each use, so that users must increase the amount of the drug in order to feel the same effects.

For more information, visit the U.S. Drug Enforcement Administration at: www.usdoj.gov/dea/ pubs/abuse/8-hallu.htm#LSD

LUNGS

The lungs are the organs that take **oxygen** into and expel carbon dioxide from the bloodstream as part of a process called respiration. Humans have two lungs, one on each side of the **heart**. The lungs are filled with tiny air sacs called alveoli that are responsible for exchanging oxygen and carbon dioxide with the **blood**.

Asthma

Asthma is a potentially life-threatening condition characterized by inflammation, constriction, and excessive **mucus** in the airways. The condition can be chronic (ever-present) or intermittent (arising occasionally,

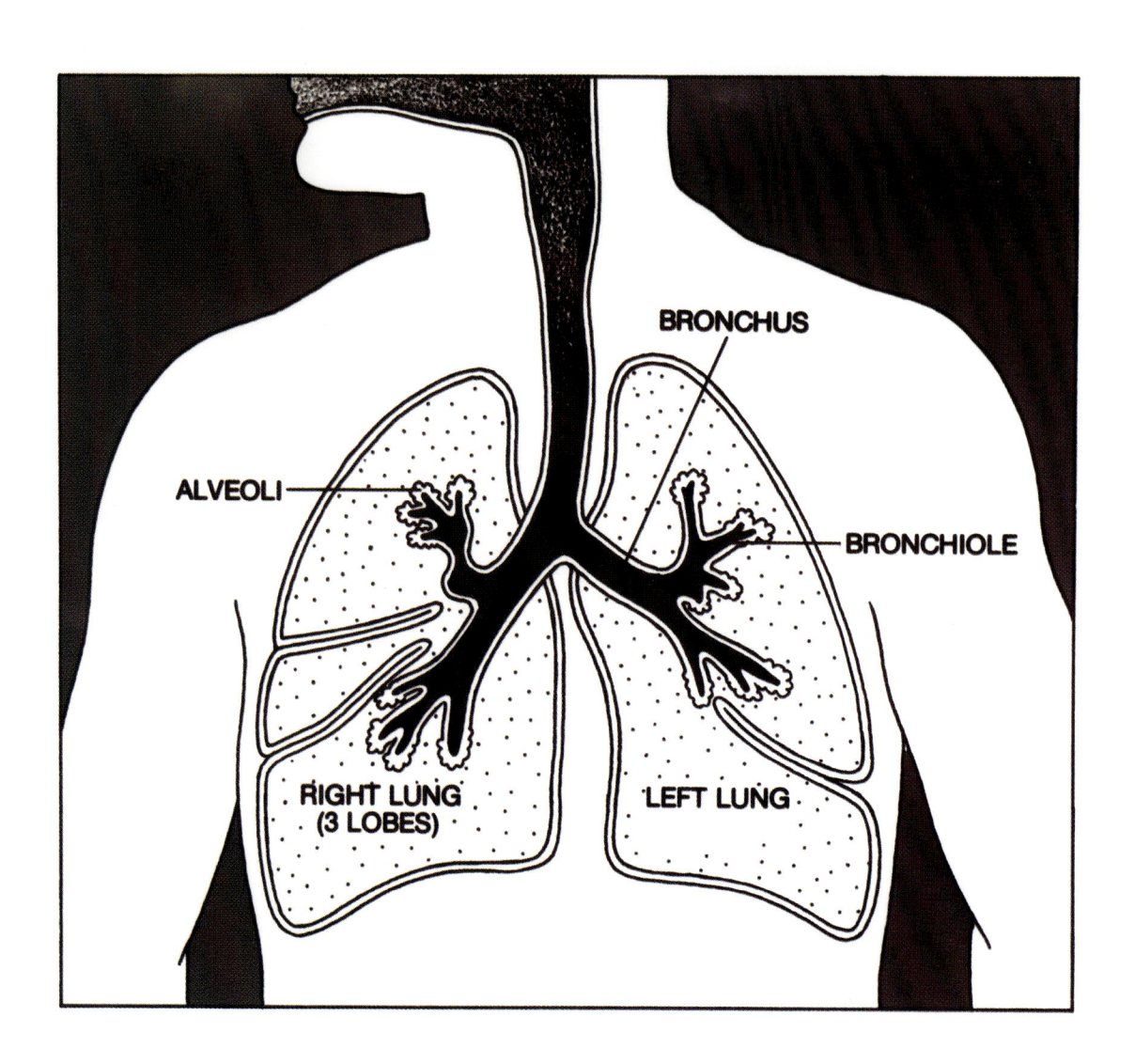

Lungs

usually in response to a specific trigger, like an *allergy*). A sudden onset of severe asthma symptoms is called an asthma attack. A person experiencing an asthma attack will have shortness of breath that may be accompanied by coughing, wheezing, increased heart rate, rapid breathing, difficulty speaking, and other symptoms. A severe asthma attack is a medical emergency that can be fatal without effective treatment.

Diagnoses of asthma have been steadily rising in recent decades. A family history of asthma is an indication of increased risk, but many cases of asthma are believed to have environmental causes, specifically, declining air quality in urban areas. Allergies commonly trigger asthma attacks, and prolonged exposure to cigarette smoke and other inhaled chemicals increases one's risk of developing asthma. Asthma cannot be cured, but the symptoms can be treated and are usually effectively managed with medications and lifestyle.

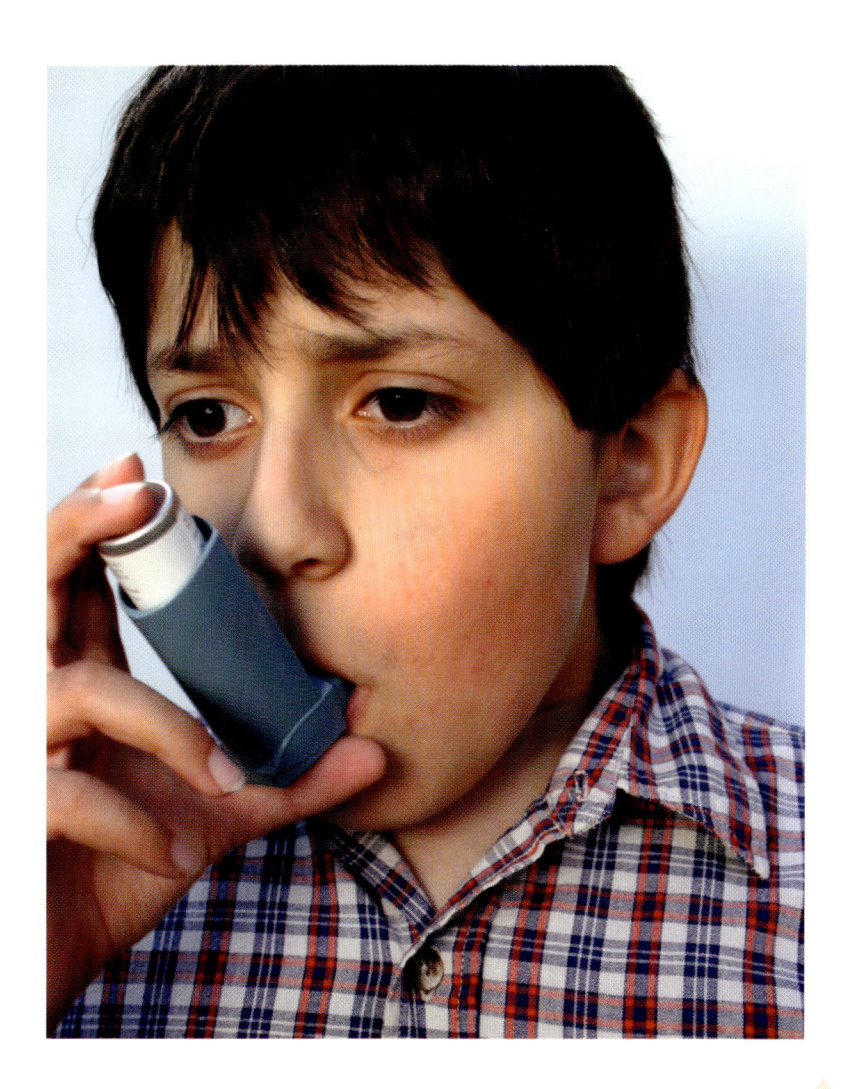

ASK THE DOCTOR

I was just diagnosed with asthma. My friend has asthma and told me I'm going to have to get rid of my dog. Is this true? I love my dog!

A: Having asthma does not automatically mean you have to get rid of your dog. Your dog may not play any role at all in your asthma, depending on whether or not you have an allergy to dog dander. Sometimes asthma is triggered by allergens, like dust, mold, pollen, or animal dander, but not all people have allergy-induced asthma. Now that you know you have asthma, one of the first things your doctor should do is give you an allergy test. This will help identify possible triggers. You should also begin paying attention to whether or not your asthma gets worse when you are around your dog. If it turns out you are in fact allergic to your dog, and your allergy is severe enough and cannot be successfully controlled with medication, you may have to think about finding it another good home. Consult with your doctor and see what your options are first.

Normally, the air you breathe travels effortlessly through your nose and mouth, down into your lungs. When a person has an asthma attack, however, the passageways become narrow, so that not as much air can get in and out.

73

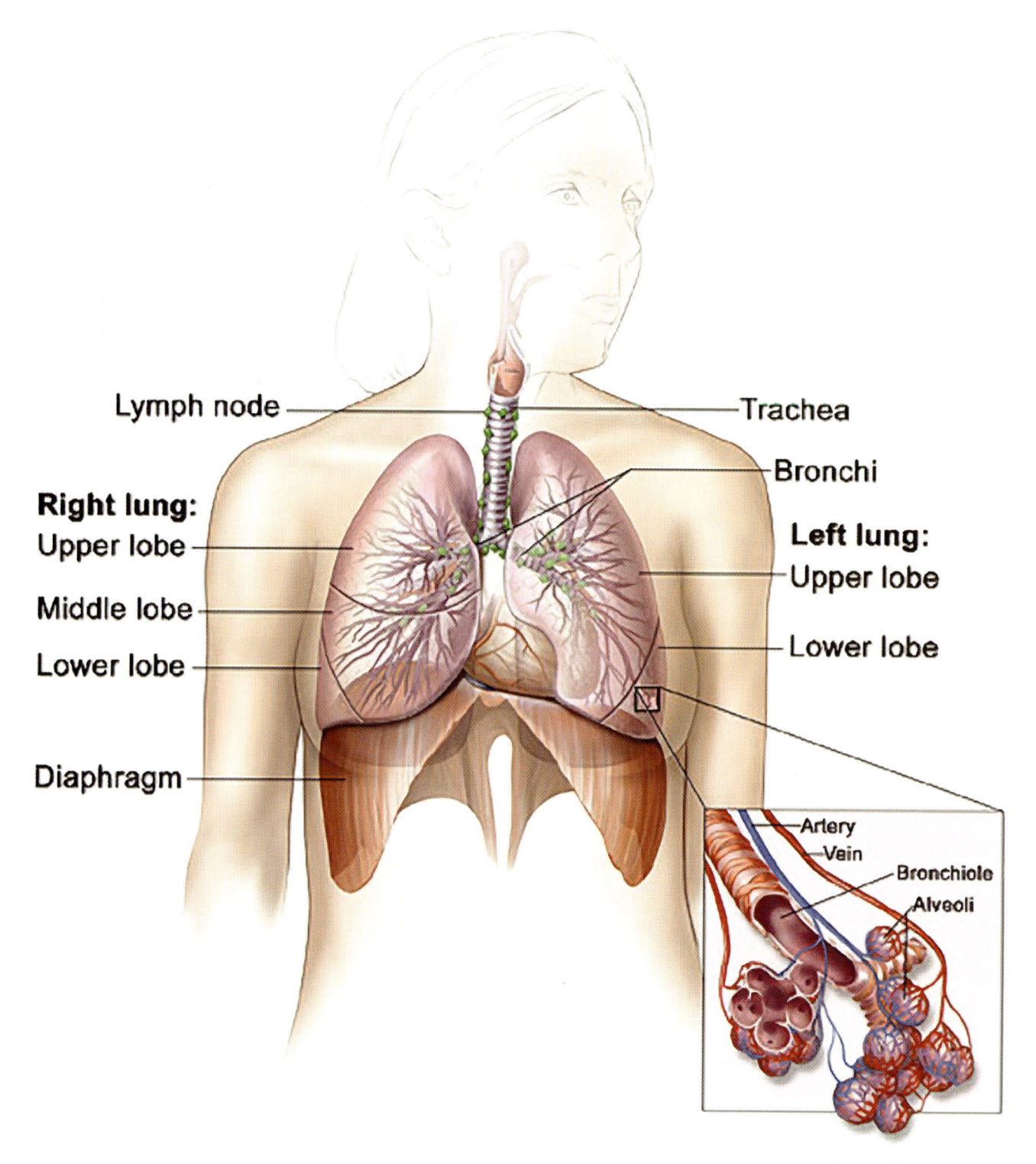

Lungs

Humans have two lungs; the left lung is divided into two lobes and the right into three lobes. Together, the lungs contain approximately 1,500 miles (2,400 km) of airways and 300 to 500 million alveoli. If you were to spread out the entire surface area of all your alveoli, they would cover roughly the same area as a tennis court—and if all the capillaries that surround your alveoli were unwound and laid end to end, they would extend for about 620 miles!

Breathing

Technically called "respiration," breathing is the act of taking air into (called inhaling) and expelling air from (called exhaling) the lungs.

Bronchitis

Bronchitis is inflammation of a set of airways in the lungs called the bronchi. This inflammation can be caused by a bacterial or viral infection, in which case it is called "acute bronchitis." There is also a long-term form of inflammation called chronic bronchitis, which is usually associated with smoking or long-term exposure to cigarette smoke. Both forms of bronchitis cause **coughing**, excess **phlegm**, shortness of breath, and wheezing.

If bronchitis is caused by a viral infection (as is true for the majority of cases), the patient must wait for the body to fight off the infection naturally. If it is bacterial, the body will also usually be able to fight off the infection on its own. Nevertheless, it is still commonplace for doctors to prescribe **antibiotics** for such infections. All people with bronchitis, regardless of the cause, should avoid cigarette smoke, allergens, and other irritants, as these may further inflame the bronchi. Bronchitis can be persistent, with the cough lasting up to a month or more. A physician should evaluate any long-lasting cough to rule out other potentially dangerous conditions.

Pulmonary Disorders

"Pulmonary disorder" is another term for any disorder of the lungs. The term pulmonary is the medical term, derived from Latin, for anything relating to the lungs.

Pulmonary disorders include these conditions:

- pulmonary embolism (a blockage in the pulmonary artery)
- pulmonary fibrosis (a form of lung disease)
- asthma
- chronic obstructive pulmonary disease (resulting in reduced airflow often as a result of long-term smoking)

Wheezing

Wheezing is a harsh, unbroken, whistling sound emanating from one's airway on expiration. It is a sign of blockage or restriction in the lower part of the airway.

LYME DISEASE

Lyme disease is a very serious bacterial infection that may be contracted from deer ticks.

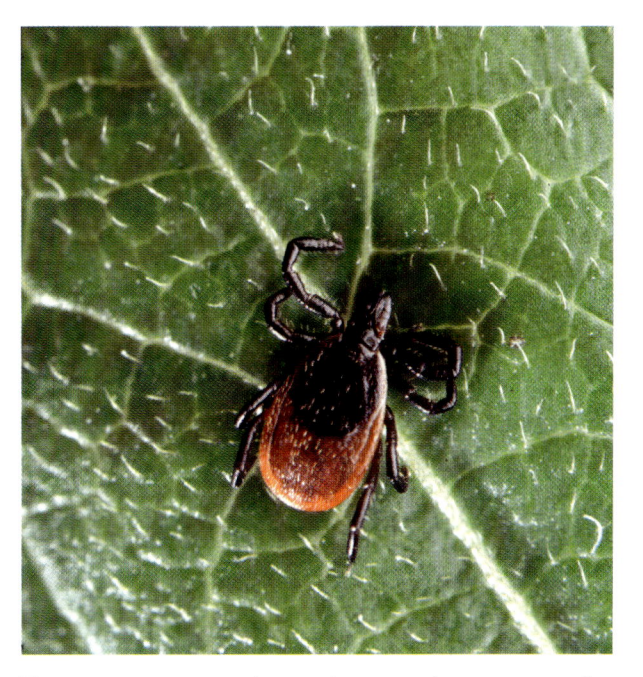

This tiny insect—a deer tick—may be carrying the bacteria that causes Lyme disease.

Lyme Disease

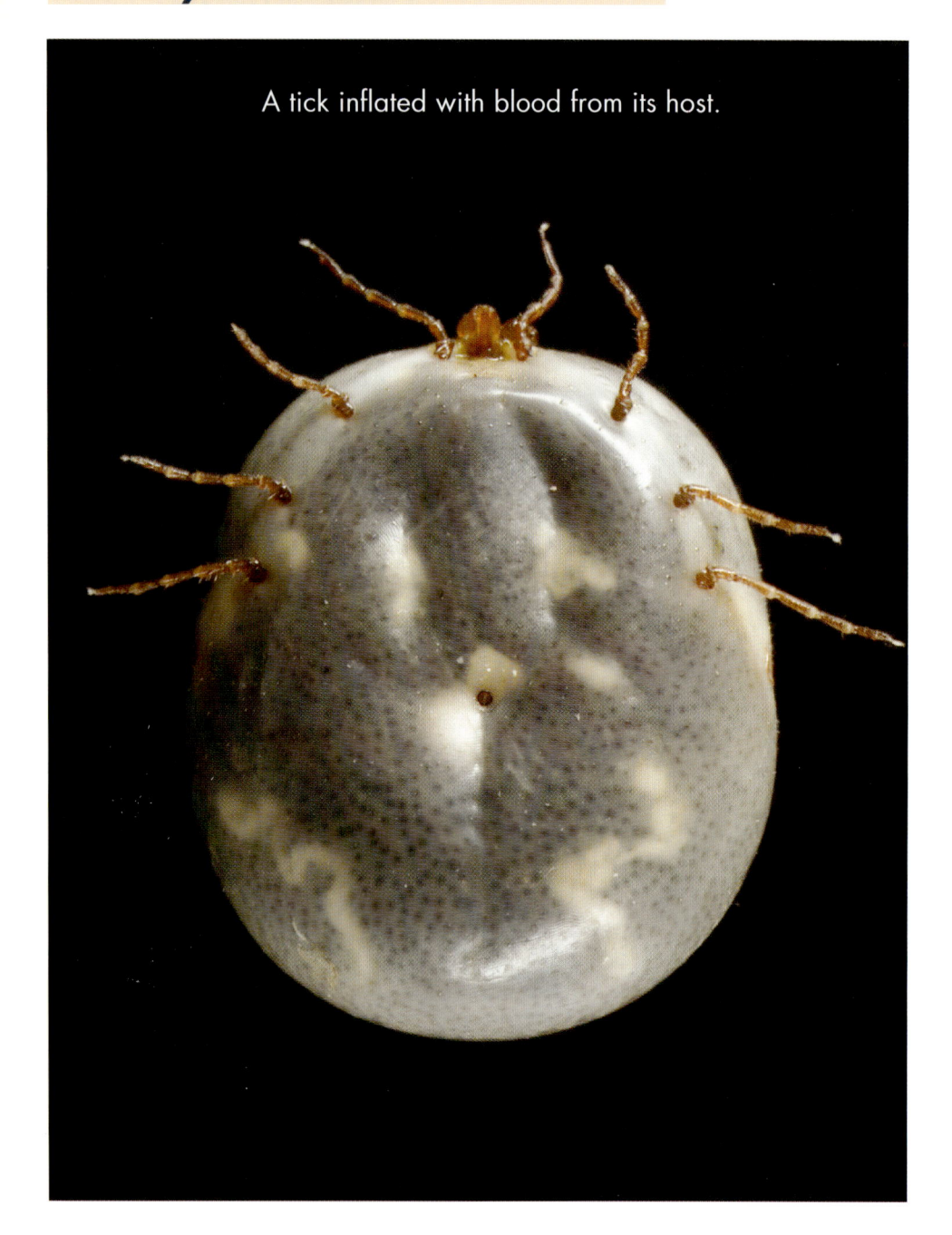

A tick inflated with blood from its host.

ASK THE DOCTOR

If I have a tick on me, how do I get rid of it?

A: There are a lot of myths about tick removal. The best way to remove a tick is carefully grab it as close to the head as possible—this is generally done with tweezers—and gently pull it out. You will want to avoid squeezing the tick's abdomen, as this can cause the tick to regurgitate into your body, increasing the risk of it transmitting bacteria to you. You will also want to try to pull out the whole tick, including the head. If the head is left behind, the area might get infected. A lot of people will tell you to burn the tick with a match or cover it with petroleum jelly to make it back out of your body. These measures usually don't work and they irritate or kill the tick, increasing the risk of it regurgitating into your system and potentially spreading disease.

Deer ticks (and some other ticks) can carry types of Borrelia bacteria, the family of **bacteria** responsible for Lyme disease. When a person becomes infected with Lyme disease, he may not have any symptoms at first. Early symptoms can include a **rash**, **fever**, and body aches. These are also the symptoms of many other illnesses, including **influenza**. For this reason, Lyme disease can be very difficult to identify, and a person may go a long time before receiving diagnosis and treatment. Delay in diagnosis and treatment greatly increases a person's chance of developing "late-stage" Lyme disease, a far more serious condition that can affect the **heart**, **nervous system**, **muscles**, **skeleton**, and even mental health.

Lyme Disease

If detected early, Lyme disease can often be effectively treated with **antibiotics**. Early detection and removal of ticks (within 24 hours of being bitten) greatly decreases the chance of becoming infected with Lyme disease or other tick-borne bacteria.

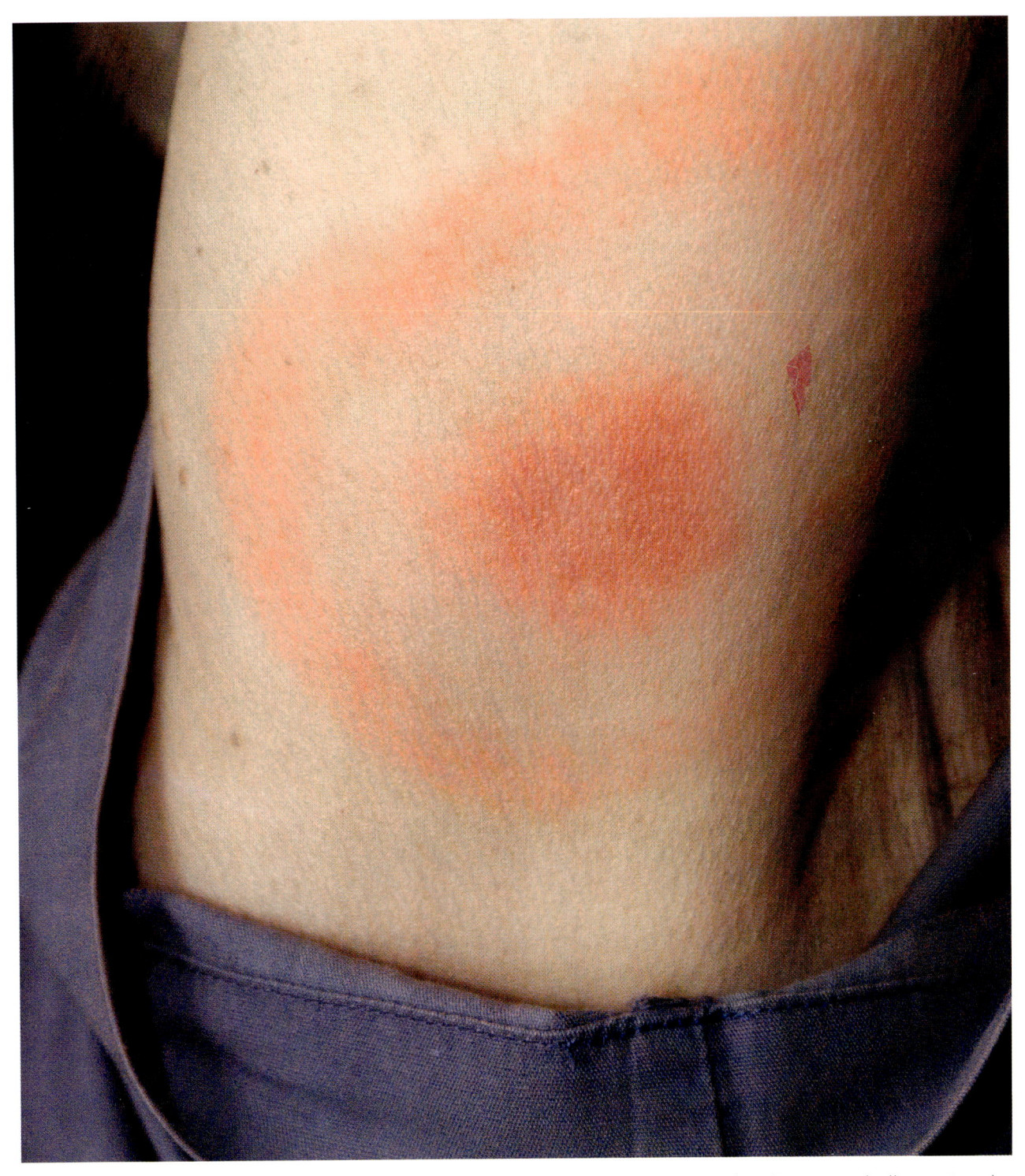

One of the most common signs of Lyme disease, and one of the earliest to develop, is a "bull's-eye" rash (shown here). Not everyone who has Lyme disease has this symptom, however.

Lymphatic System

LYMPHATIC SYSTEM

The lymphatic system is a "secondary" circulatory system of the body. Like the primary **circulatory system**, the lymphatic system is composed of a network of vessels through which fluid flows. The lymphatic system is an important part of the **immune system**. It contains large collections of white blood cells, and one of its major jobs is to filter **bacteria**, **viruses**, and other harmful entities out of the body. The lymphatic system, however, has other jobs as well, including transporting **fat** and collecting extra fluid from the body. Malfunction of the lymph system can result in edema, the build up of fluid in the body's tissues.

Lacteals

The lacteals are a specific type of lymph vessel. They are located in the small intestine. Their job is to absorb fats, which are important nutrients, from the small intestine into the lymph fluid.

Lymph Ducts

Lymph ducts are large lymphatic vessels that collect lymph fluid from an area of the body and return it to the circulatory system. The human body has two lymph ducts. The largest is the thoracic duct. Most of the body's lymph fluid drains into this duct. There is also the right lymphatic duct, which drains lymph fluid from the right arm and chest and the right side of the head and neck.

Lymph Fluid

Lymph fluid is the liquid component of the lymphatic system. It bathes the body's tissues and circulates through the lymphatic system collecting excess fluids, retrieving fats from the intestines and delivering them to the circulatory system, and bringing pathogens into the lymph nodes where they can be destroyed. Unlike blood, which is pumped by the heart, lymph fluid is not moved around the body through the

---

ASK THE DOCTOR

I have a sore lump behind my earlobe and another on my throat just beneath my jaw. They've been there for more than 2 weeks. Could they be tumors?

A: It is unlikely that they are tumors. These are common locations for detecting swollen lymph nodes, and sometimes these lymph nodes can take a long time to return to their normal size after an illness or infection. However, 2 weeks is a long time for lymph nodes to remain swollen, and I typically recommend that, after 2 weeks, a doctor examine the swelling. Even if they are not tumors, lymph nodes that remain swollen for a long time can be a sign of another problem, including a persistent or more serious infection, such as mononucleosis.

DID YOU KNOW?

Lymph is a clear-to-white fluid made of red blood cells; proteins and fats from the intestines called chyle; and white blood cells, especially lymphocytes, the cells that attack bacteria in the blood.

Lymphatic System

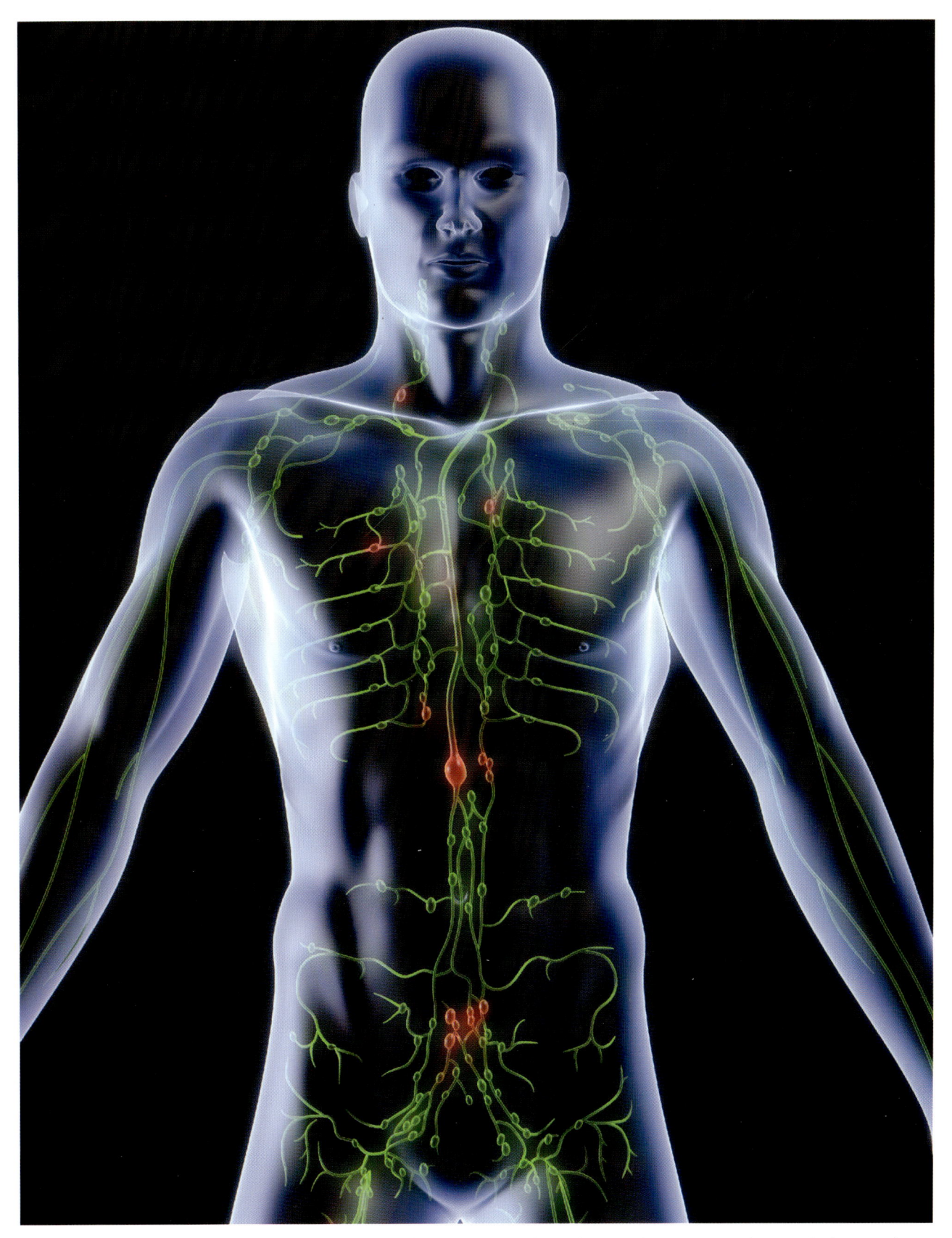

When bacteria are recognized in the lymph fluid, the lymph nodes produce more infection-fighting white blood cells, which causes the nodes to swell.

Lymphatic System

pumping action of an organ. Instead, it flows mostly due to the movements of tiny muscles that rhythmically contract, helping to push the lymph fluid around the body.

Lymph Nodes

The lymphatic system contains approximately 500 to 600 lymph nodes, also commonly called glands. These nodes are located all over the body, but they are particularly concentrated in the neck, armpits and underside of the upper arms, the right side of the chest, and the groin area. These nodes are part of the body's filtration system. They are filled with white blood cells. They also have a structure that traps **pathogens** inside the node, where they are destroyed by the white blood cells.

Some lymph nodes are very small, just a few fractions of an inch, while others are quite large, reaching an inch or slightly larger across. Some larger lymph nodes can be felt by hand, especially in the neck. Lymph nodes may become more noticeable when infected, because they usually swell and may become sore. It is quite common for a person to suddenly notice a lump on her body that wasn't there before. If this lump is in the neck, underarms, or groin, it is very likely a swollen lymph node. This usually means that an infection is or recently was present in the body, even if the person never actually felt sick. Once the infection has been fought off, the lymph node will shrink back to its normal size.

Lymph nodes are also a fairly common site for **tumors** and **cancer**. This can also cause an enlarged lymph node. In the case of tumors or cancer, the enlarged lymph node is usually painless. A doctor should evaluate any lump that does not disappear after a few days or weeks. In the case of lumps found

Your lymph system extends through your entire body, supporting the work of your circulatory system. As your blood circulates, fluid leaks into the body tissues, carrying food to the cells. The leaked fluid then drains into the lymph vessels and is carried through the lymph vessels to the base of the neck, where it is emptied back into the bloodstream. This circulation of fluid through the body is going on all the time.

in the **breasts** or **testicles**, one should seek immediate medical evaluation as soon as the lump is discovered. This is to rule out the possibility of breast or testicular cancers, cancers for which early detection greatly increases long-term survival.

Lymph Vessels

Lymph vessels are the tubes that carry lymph fluid all over the body. Lymph vessels have valves that permit the lymph fluid to flow in only one direction. Small muscles help push the lymph fluid through the lymph vessels. Fluids that leak from the primary circulatory system eventually drain into the lymph system, where they are carried by lymph vessels and ultimately returned to circulation. Lymph capillaries are a type of lymph vessel.

Lymphatic Tissue

Lymphatic tissue is a type of tissue found throughout the lymph system that is very high in white blood cells. Some parts of the body that are important to immune functioning contain a large amount of lymphatic tissue. These include the **spleen** (the organ responsible for filtering and destroying old and damaged red blood cells), the thymus (an organ responsible for producing certain types of white blood cells), and the tonsils (masses of tissue in the throat responsible for helping to fight infection, especially infections of the upper-respiratory system).

Glossary of Health Terms

adolescent health: The branch of health care providing services to people generally between the ages of 13 and 18.

anatomy: The study of the structure of the body.

autoimmune diseases: Illnesses resulting from a person's own immune system attacking his or her body.

bioterrorism: The use of biological agents, such as pathogens, to inspire fear for political purposes.

cardiovascular: Referring to the part of the circulatory system made up of the heart and blood vessels.

CDC: Centers for Disease Control and Prevention; organization that aims to prevent disease and improve health in the United States.

children's health: Health care dealing with the well-being of infants, children, and adolescents.

chronic disease: An illness lasting for longer than 3 months.

clinical trials: Research studies aimed at determining how humans react to new drugs or procedures.

communicable diseases: Contagious diseases; illnesses that can be transmitted from person to person.

controlled substances: A drug whose sale or use has been declared illegal by law, except in cases of a doctor's prescription.

CPR: cardiopulmonary resuscitation; Lifesaving procedure performed when a person's heart or lungs have stopped working.

Department of Health and Human Services: DHHS; the main U.S. agency that addresses health concerns—includes the FDA, the CDC, and the NIH.

DNA: deoxyribonucleic acid; a molecule that is the basis for human genetic information.

Glossary of Health Terms

DSM-IV: *Diagnostic and Statistical Manual of Mental Disorders;* the most current edition of a classification of psychiatric disorders.

diagnostics: The practice of identifying a disease by its symptoms.

disorder: An abnormal physical or mental condition.

drug: A substance used as medicine to treat illness; also, a chemical substance used for recreational purposes because of its effects on behavior.

drug schedules: System set up by the Controlled Substances Act of 1970 that classifies drugs according to their medicinal properties and potential for abuse.

emergency care: Treatment given when immediate attention is necessary.

environmental health: Addresses health factors that are determined by the environment, such as the spread of disease.

epidemics: Diseases that spread over a wide geographic area and affect a large number of people.

epidemiology: The study of the cause, spread, and control of disease.

family health: Medical branch that deals with the health of family units and individuals within families.

fitness: The condition of being physically healthy, especially because of good nutrition and exercise.

FDA: Food and Drug Administration: U. S. agency that oversees products that affect consumers' health, such as food, cosmetics, and drugs.

food safety: Refers to the maintenance of food quality to prevent disease.

global health: Health issues that concern people across countries' borders.

health care: Services provided for by medical professionals to prevent and treat illness.

health care workers: People who work to address health issues; includes physicians, nurses, surgeons, and pharmacists.

health insurance: A means of paying money to guarantee being able to pay for treatment of future health problems.

HMO: Health Maintenance Organization; an organization that provides medical care based on a prepaid contract.

health occupations: Jobs dealing with health care.

herd immunity: The resistance of a large group of people to a specific disease because most individuals within the group are immune.

Glossary of Health Terms

immunity: Resistance to a disease because of genes, a vaccination, or previous infection.
injury: Accidental or purposeful damage done to the body.

LGBT: Acronym referring to lesbian, gay, bisexual, and transgender people.
life expectancy: Number of years a person is expected to live, based on lifestyle and environment.

Medicaid: U.S. public programs that give health care to those who cannot afford to pay for it.
Medicare: U.S. public health insurance coverage for senior citizens and some people with disabilities.
mental health: A person's emotional and psychological condition, and the branch of medicine that addresses this.

NIDA: National Institute of Drug Abuse; part of NIH that conducts research on drug abuse with the goal of preventing and treating addiction.
NIH: National Institutes of Health; research-oriented U. S. health agency made up of several separate institutes.
NSAIDs: Nonsteroidal anti-inflammatory drugs; used to treat illnesses causing inflammation, such as arthritis.

occupational hazards: Job conditions that put a person at risk for injury or illness.
opportunistic infections: Infections that develop because of a weakened immune system.
OTC drugs: Over-the-counter drugs; medicines sold without a prescription.

pathology: The study of disease.
patient safety: The prevention of accidental injury because of a medical error.
pharmaceutical: Relating to medicinal drugs, also known as pharmaceutical products.
physiology: The study of the function of living things.
primary care physician: PCP; the doctor, usually a family physician or pediatrician, who provides individuals with primary care.
primary health care: Basic, regular health services that serve as the starting point for other, more specific health care.

research: Scientific investigation.
RNA: ribonucleic acid; a molecule in cells that works with DNA to produce proteins.

Glossary of Health Terms

safety: Avoiding the risk of harm or injury.

SAMHSA: Substance Abuse and Mental Health Services Administration; part of the U.S. Public Health Services that aims to prevent and treat drug abuse, as well as to improve mental health services.

sanitation: Measures taken to protect health, especially relating to waste disposal.

substance abuse: The overuse of a substance, such as a drug, for non-medical purposes.

teen health: The branch of health care that addresses issues specifically related to teenagers, such as nutrition, drugs, and sexual activity.

terminal illness: A disease that will lead to death.

traveler's health: Relating to the prevention of diseases or conditions a person may acquire while traveling.

vehicle safety: The prevention of injury due to automobiles.

women's health: Addresses women's health issues such as reproduction, but also women's responses to non-gender-specific conditions.

WHO: World Health Organization; United Nations (UN) agency meant to improve global health conditions.

Learn More

Birth Defects
Centers for Disease Control and Prevention–Birth Defects
www.cdc.gov/ncbddd/bd/facts.htm

Cleft Palate Foundation
www.cleftline.org

Foundation for Faces of Children
www.facesofchildren.org/conditions/cleft_palate.htm

The Body
Brain Atlas
www.brainexplorer.org/brain_atlas/Brainatlas_index.shtml

National Eye Institute–Cornea
www.nei.nih.gov/health/cornealdisease/index.asp#b1

National Kidney Foundation
www.kidney.org

Partners in Assistive Technology Training and Services–Skeletal System
www.webschoolsolutions.com/patts/systems/skeleton.htm

Society for Neuroscience–Biological Clocks
www.sfn.org/index.cfm?pagename=brainBriefings_biologicalClocks

Womenshealth.org–Varicose Veins
www.4woman.gov/faq/varicose.htm

Diseases and Disorders
American Academy of Dermatology–Skin Cancer
www.aad.org/public

American Cancer Society
www.cancer.org/docroot/CRI/content/CRI_2_4_1x_What_Is_Cancer_72.asp?sitearea=CRI

American Diabetes Association
www.diabetes.org/about-diabetes.jsp

American Gastroenterological Association–Cirrhosis
www.gastro.org/wmspage.cfm?parm1=681

Learn More

American Headache Society
www.achenet.org

BreastCancer.org
www.breastcancer.org

Celiac Disease Foundation
www.celiac.org/cd-main.php

Centers for Disease Control and Prevention–HIV
www.cdc.gov/hiv/resources/qa/qa1.htm

Centers for Disease Control and Prevention–Meningitis
www.cdc.gov/ncidod/dbmd/diseaseinfo/meningococcal_g.htm

Christopher and Dana Reeve Foundation–Paralysis
www.christopherreeve.org/site/c.gelMLPOpGjF/b.899265/k.CC03/Home.htm

DermWeb–Psoriasis
www.dermatology.org/skincare/psoriasis/psorhand.html

Macular Degeneration Network
www.macular-degeneration.org

Malaria Site
www.malariasite.com/malaria/WhatIsMalaria.htm

Mayo Clinic–Back Pain
www.mayoclinic.com/health/back-pain/DS00171/DSECTION=8

Mayo Clinic–Tuberculosis
www.mayoclinic.com/health/tuberculosis/DS00372/DSECTION=1

MedicineNet.com–Allergies
www.medicinenet.com/allergies/focus.htm

MedicineNet.com–Syncope
www.medterms.com/script/main/art.asp?articlekey=5612

MedlinePlus–Incontinence
www.nlm.nih.gov/medlineplus/ency/article/001270.htm

Muscular Dystrophy Association
www.mdausa.org

National Cancer Institute–Breast Cancer
www.cancer.gov/cancertopics/pdq/screening/breast/Patient/page2

Learn More

National Digestive Diseases Information Clearinghouse–Crohn's Disease
www.digestive.niddk.nih.gov/ddiseases/pubs/crohns_ez/index.htm

National Heart, Lung, and Blood Institute–Asthma
www.nhlbi.nih.gov/health/dci/Diseases/Asthma/Asthma_WhatIs.html

National Institute on Deafness and Other Communication Disorders
www.nidcd.nih.gov

National Multiple-Sclerosis Society
www.nationalmssociety.org/site/PageServer?pagename=HOM_ABOUT_homepage

National Osteoporosis Foundation
www.nof.org/osteoporosis

National Parkinson Foundation
www.parkinson.org/NETCOMMUNITY/Page.aspx?pid=201&srcid=-2

Parkinson's Disease Foundation
www.pdf.org

Womenshealth.org–Pelvic Inflammatory Disease
www.womenshealth.gov/faq/stdpids.htm

Drug Abuse
eMedicineHealth–Overdose
www.emedicinehealth.com/drug_overdose/article_em.htm

National Institute on Drug Abuse
www.nida.nih.gov

Palo Alto Medical Foundation–Alcohol Abuse
www.pamf.org/teen/healthinfo/index.cfm?section=healthinfo&page=article&sgml_id=hw130547

Environmental Health
Centers for Disease Control and Prevention–Parasites
www.cdc.gov/ncidod/dpd/aboutparasites.htm

Environmental Protection Agency–Airnow.gov
www.epa.gov/airnow/airaware/day1.html

Health Care
American Dental Association
www.ada.org

Children's Hospital Boston–Neonatal Intensive Care Unit
www.childrenshospital.org/az/Site1736/mainpageS1736P0.html

Learn More

March of Dimes–Prenatal Care
www.marchofdimes.com/pnhec/159_513.asp

National Family Caregivers Association
www.thefamilycaregiver.org/improving_caregiving

WebMD–Chiropractics
www.webmd.com/back-pain/guide/chiropractic-care-and-back-pain

Mental Health
Autism Society of America
www.autism-society.org/site/PageServer

Bipolar.com
www.bipolar.com/index.html

Bipolar Help Center
www.bipolarhelpcenter.com/index.jsp?reqNavId=0

Centers for Disease Control and Prevention and Prevention–ADHD
www.cdc.gov/ncbddd/adhd/what.htm

The Cleveland Clinic–Munchausen Syndrome
www.clevelandclinic.org/health/healthinfo/docs/2800/2821.asp?index=9833

Mayo Clinic
www.mayoclinic.com/health/mental-illness/HQ01079/UPDATEAPP=0

National Institute of Mental Health–Depression
www.nimh.nih.gov/health/topics/depression/index.shtml

Obsessive Compulsive Foundation
www.ocfoundation.org

Penn State Children's Hospital–Mental Retardation
www.hmc.psu.edu/childrens/healthinfo/m/mentalretardation.htm

Postpartum Support International
www.postpartum.net

Psychology Today–Multiple Personality Disorder
www.psychologytoday.com/conditions/did.html

University of Maryland Medical Center–Eating Disorders
www.umm.edu/patiented/articles/what_causes_eating_disorders_000049_3.htm
U.S. Department of Veterans Affairs–Posttraumatic Stress Disorder
www.ncptsd.va.gov/ncmain/index.jsp

Learn More

Nutrition

American Heart Association–Cholesterol
www.americanheart.org/presenter.jhtml?identifier=3046103

Answers.com–Basal Metabolic Rate
www.answers.com/topic/basal-metabolic-rate?cat=health

Centers for Disease Control and Prevention–Obesity
www.cdc.gov/nccdphp/dnpa/obesity

MERCK–Calcium
www.merck.com/mmhe/sec12/ch155/ch155b.html

Plastic Surgery

American Society of Plastic Surgeons
www.plasticsurgery.org/patients_consumers/procedures

Reproduction

American Academy of Family Physicians–Premature Babies
www.familydoctor.org/online/famdocen/home/children/parents/infants/283.html

The American College of Obstetricians and Gynecologists–Miscarriage
www.acog.org/publications/patient_education/bp090.cfm

Centers for Disease Control and Prevention–Breastfeeding
www.cdc.gov/breastfeeding

MedicineNet.com–Condoms
www.medicinenet.com/condoms/article.htm

MedicineNet.com–Menopause
www.medicinenet.com/menopause/article.htm

MedicineNet.com–Oral Contraceptives
www.medicinenet.com/oral_contraceptives_birth_control_pills/article.htm

University of Pennsylvania Health System–Multiple Births
www.pennhealth.com/health_info/pregnancy/000199.htm

Womenshealth.org–PMS
www.4woman.gov/faq/pms.htm

Travel Health

Centers for Disease Control and Prevention–Motion Sickness
wwwn.cdc.gov/travel/yellowBookCh6-MotionSickness.aspx

Centers for Disease Control and Prevention–Traveler's Health
wwwn.cdc.gov/travel/default.aspx

Learn More

Treatment and Prevention

American Chiropractic Association–Posture
www.amerchiro.org/content_css.cfm?CID=1452

Centers for Disease Control and Prevention–Mumps Vaccination
www.cdc.gov/vaccines/vpd-vac/mumps/default.htm

LA Fire Department–Accident Preparedness
www.preparedness.info/npi/accprev/default.htm

Medpage Today–HPV Test
www.medpagetoday.com/HematologyOncology/OtherCancers/dh/3082

National Cancer Institute–Cancer Treatment
www.cancer.gov/cancerinfo/treatment

National Cancer Institute–Mammography
www.cancer.gov/newscenter/pressreleases/DMISTQandA

NeurosurgeryToday.org
www.neurosurgerytoday.org/what/usa/neurosurgeons.asp

Transplant Living
www.transplantliving.org/beforethetransplant/qa.aspx

WebMD–Contacts
www.webmd.com/eye-health/contact-lenses

Index

abdomen 35, 36
AIDS 14, 22
alcohol 32, 34, 37, 38, 39
allergen 12, 73, 75
allergies 12, 13, 16, 20, 73
Alzheimer's disease 20
anesthetics 31, 68
antibiotic 51, 77
anus 18, 36
anxiety 18
appetite 32, 47, 72
arthritis 14, 15, 42, 44, 45, 48, 68
asthma 72, 73, 75
autoimmune disorders 13, 14, 15

back 46, 68
bacteria 12, 20, 21, 22, 37, 50, 51, 75, 76, 77, 78
bile 43, 66
binge drinking 38, 39
birth 15, 18, 19, 25, 34, 41, 63, 67
  multiple 39
bladder 19, 20, 47
  gallbladder 36, 66
blood 12, 24, 25, 34, 38, 46, 47, 57, 59, 61, 72, 78
  cells 12, 41, 57, 58, 59, 66, 67, 78, 80, 81
  flow 12
  infection 22
  pressure 72
  stream 12, 28, 32, 35, 36, 60, 72
  test 27, 59
  vessels 11, 31, 52
Blood Alcohol Concentration (BAC) 38
bone 40, 42, 43, 44, 47, 48, 57, 59, 64
  marrow 59, 61, 62
bowels 18, 37, 39, 53, 54
brain 12, 32, 37, 39, 55
breastfeeding 25, 49
breasts 81
breathing 73, 75
bronchitis 75

caffeine 34, 39, 54
cancer 9, 14, 36, 37, 57, 58, 59, 60, 61, 62, 80, 81
  laryngeal 50
  precancerous 13, 36
  stomach 20
cartilage 42
celiac disease 37
cells 11, 12, 13, 14, 15, 24, 57, 58, 60, 61
  blood 12, 41, 47, 57, 58, 59, 60, 66, 67, 78, 80, 81
  cancer 14, 60, 61, 62
Centers for Disease Control 17, 38
cervix 35
circulatory system 78, 81
cirrhosis 66, 67
collagen 65
colon 36, 54
common cold 27

Index

congenital 15
constipation 37
Controlled Substances Act 33
cornea 53
cough 19, 22, 23, 28, 29, 30, 50, 73, 75
Crohn's disease 37
cuts 11, 49, 52

death 14, 17, 32, 38, 39, 60
depression 32
diabetes 34, 35, 47
dialysis 47
diarrhea 18, 37
diet 8, 18, 34, 37, 39, 47, 54
digestion 66
   conditions 20
   system 39, 54
   tract 20, 36
disability 14, 16, 17, 54, 55, 56
dislocation 44, 65
drugs
   medicinal 30, 59, 62, 70, 72
   recreational 31
dyslexia 56

eggs 39
erectile dysfunction 17, 18
erection 18
exercise 18, 19, 20, 34, 43
eyes 41, 52, 53, 67

face 8, 13, 14, 32
fallopian tubes 35
fat 36, 39, 47, 65, 78
fatigue 18, 26, 27, 47, 60, 62
fever 27, 28, 30, 31, 59, 76
fiber 37, 39, 53, 54
fungus 22, 23

gastroenteritis 31
gastrointestinal tract 24, 30, 31
genetic 8, 15, 59
glands 36, 49, 65

hallucinations 32, 40, 72
hallucinogens 70
headache 28
heart 14, 32, 72, 77, 78
   burn 20, 51
   rate 72, 73
hepatitis 67
herpes 22, 24, 26

hip 43, 45
HIV 15, 25
hormones 15, 18, 47
hygiene 30

immune system 11, 12, 13, 14, 15, 16, 21, 22, 26, 28, 59, 62, 78
immunization 16, 17
immunodeficiency 14, 15, 16
impotence 17, 18
in vitro fertilization 39
incontinence 18, 19, 20
indigestion 20
infection 12, 13, 14, 15, 16, 17, 19, 20, 21, 22, 24, 25, 27, 29, 30, 31, 37, 39, 40, 50, 51, 52, 59, 62, 75, 78, 80, 81
   airborne transmission 22, 23
   droplet transmission 23, 24
   fecal-oral transmission 24
   horizontal transmission 24
   indirect contact 24
   infectious disease transmission 22
   vector-borne transmission 25
   vertical transmission 25
infertility 28
inflammation 12, 15, 20, 28, 50, 67, 72, 75
influenza (flu) 22, 27, 28, 29, 30, 31, 73
inhalants 31, 32, 33
insomnia 33, 34
insulin 34, 35
internal examination 35, 54
intestines 36, 37, 78
   large 36, 37, 54
   small 36, 66, 78
intoxication 32, 37, 38
irritable bowel syndrome 37, 39
itches 39, 40

jaundice 41, 67, 68
joints 14, 15, 42, 43, 44, 45, 48, 59, 64, 65

kidneys 14, 32, 46, 47, 48
knees 43, 44, 45, 48

lacerations 49
lacteals 78
laryngitis 50, 51
larynx 50, 51
lasers 51, 52, 53
laxatives 39, 53, 54
lead poisoning 54
leukemia 57, 58, 59, 62

Index

life expectancy 63, 64
ligaments 42, 44, 64, 65
liposuction 65
liver 14, 32, 36, 41, 65, 66, 67, 68
LSD 31, 70, 72
lungs 14, 22, 28, 32, 34, 50, 72, 73, 75
lupus 14, 15
Lyme disease 25, 75, 76, 77
lymph
   fluid 78, 80, 81
   nodes 27, 59, 78, 80
   system 78, 81
   vessels 80, 81

malaria 17, 22, 25
malnutrition 15
minerals 36, 37, 47
mononucleosis 26, 27, 28, 78
mucus 11, 23, 29, 31, 36, 41, 72
multiple sclerosis 20
muscle 18, 19, 20, 28, 31, 36, 47, 77, 81

National Institute of Alcohol Abuse and Alcoholism (NIAA) 38
nausea 30, 31, 32, 47, 60
neck 20, 50, 78, 80
nerves 18, 19
   nerve damage 18, 20
nervous system 32, 77
nitrites 31, 32
nose 11, 23, 30

obesity 34, 43, 44, 45
osteoarthritis 68
ovaries 35
oxygen 28, 72

pain 14, 15, 20, 31, 39, 40, 44
   back 68
   joint 43, 45
   medication 47
painkiller 51
pancreas 34, 36
pandemic 28, 29, 30
pap test 35
paralysis 20
parasites 21, 22, 25
Parkinson's disease 20
pathogens 11, 12, 13, 16, 20, 21, 22, 23, 24, 25, 78, 80
pelvic exam 35
phlegm 75

pneumonia 28
pregnancy 9, 19, 25, 34, 39
   multiple birth 39
prostrate 19
protein 36, 47
pulmonary disorders 75

rash 14, 23, 39, 76
rectum 18, 35, 37
reproductive system 28, 35
respiratory
   droplets 23
   fluid 23
   infection 22
   system 28, 31, 81
rheumatoid arthritis 14, 15, 68

saliva 27, 29
sexually transmitted infections (STIs) 24, 39
skin 11, 13, 14, 23, 24, 39, 40, 41, 49, 59, 67
skull 42, 49
sleep 33, 34, 62
smallpox 17
sneeze 19, 22, 23, 29, 30
sore throat 27, 28, 50
sperm 39
spleen 27, 81
STDs 9, 24
stem cells 61
stitches 49
stomach 20, 30, 31, 36, 50, 51, 66
stress 13, 14, 15, 18, 19, 20, 33, 34, 39, 62, 63
stroke 20
surgery 18, 19, 45, 65
   cosmetic 52
   LASIK 53

testicles 81
therapy
   biological 62
   chemotherapy 59, 61
   light 41
   phototherapy 68
   physical 45
   radiation 59, 60
   relaxation 34
tissue 11, 13, 14, 15, 16, 28, 35, 36, 42, 44, 45, 49, 51, 52, 57, 64, 65, 66, 67, 78, 81
transplant 16, 22, 47, 48, 59, 61, 66, 67
tuberculosis 22
tumor 22, 52, 78, 80

Index

urine 18, 19, 20, 46, 47
uterus 19, 35, 39

vaccination 16
vagina 18, 24, 35
virus 11, 12, 14, 21, 22, 23, 24, 25, 26, 27, 28, 29, 30, 51, 67, 78

vitamins 36, 47
vitiligo 13, 14, 15
vocal cords 50, 51

weight 20, 32, 43, 44, 48, 54
wheezing 73, 75
World Health Organization 8, 17

Author Biography

Elise DeVore Berlan, MD, MPH, FAAP, is a faculty member of the Division of Adolescent Health at Nationwide Children's Hospital and an Assistant Professor of Clinical Pediatrics at The Ohio State University College of Medicine. She completed her Fellowship in Adolescent Medicine at Children's Hospital Boston and obtained a Master's Degree in Public Health at the Harvard School of Public Health. Dr. Berlan completed her residency in pediatrics at the Children's Hospital of Philadelphia, where she also served an additional year as Chief Resident. She received her medical degree from the University of Iowa College of Medicine. Dr. Berlan is board certified in Pediatrics and board eligible in Adolescent Medicine. She provides primary care and consultative services in the area of Young Women's Health, including gynecological problems, concerns about puberty, reproductive health services, and reproductive endocrine disorders.

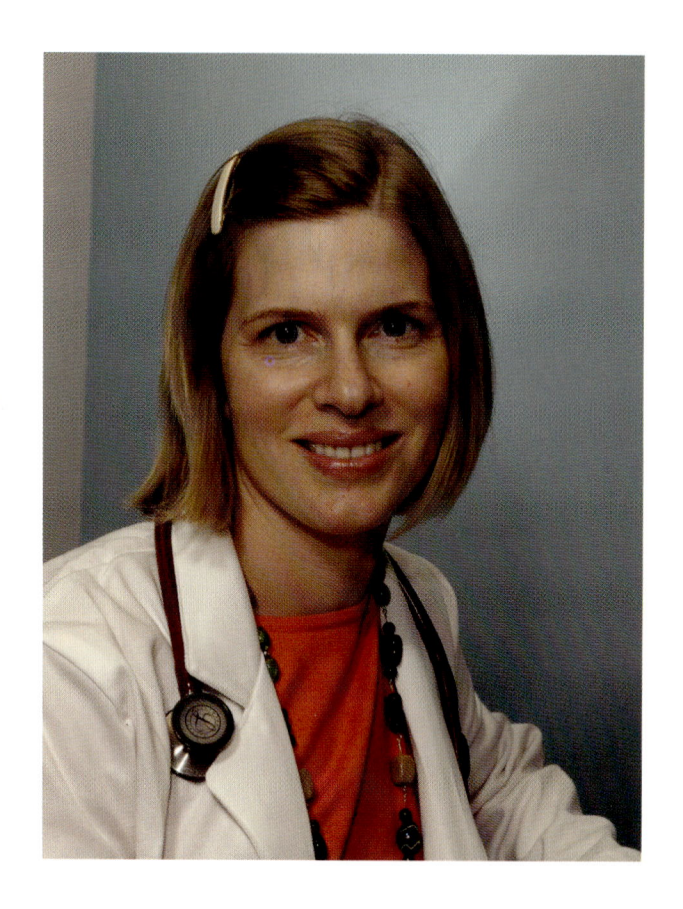